Ketogenic Diet Cookbook

The Best Way To Revitalize Yourself And Detox Your Body This Year

By

Stacey Bell

Table of Contents

Keto Dessert & Chaffle Cookbook 2021 with Pictures

Intermittent Fasting for Women Over 60

Gourmet Keto Diet Cookbook For Women After 50

The 15-Day Keto Fasting Cookbook

Keto diet Cookbook

Keto Dessert & Chaffle Cookbook 2021 with Pictures

Quick and Easy, Sugar-Low Bombs, Chaffle and Cakes Recipes to Shed Weight, Boost Your Mood and Live Ketogenic lifestyle

By

Stacey Bell

Table of Contents

Introduction

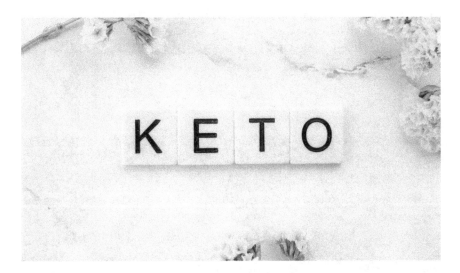

The ketogenic diet or Keto is a low-carbohydrate, mild protein, high-fat diet that will help you lose fat more efficiently. It has several advantages for weight reduction, wellbeing, and efficiency, so a rising number of healthcare professionals & practitioners recommend it.

Fat as a form of nutrition

For nutrition, the body uses three fuel sources: carbohydrates, fats and proteins. Carbohydrates convert into blood sugar or glucose in the bloodstream and are the primary fuel source for the body. If carbohydrates are not accessible, your body then depends on fat as an energy source. Protein is the primary building block of muscles and tissues. Protein could also be processed into glucose in a pinch and utilized for energy.

The keto diet encourages your body to utilize fat as the primary source of nutrition instead of carbohydrates, a ketosis mechanism. You consume too little carbs on the keto diet that the body cannot depend on glucose for nutrition. And your body turns to utilize fat for energy rather than carbs, as keto foods are filled with fat. A major part of the calories, almost 70 to 80% come from fat, consuming 15 to 20% of calories from protein and barely 5% calories from carbohydrates (that makes for about 20 to 30 grams of carbohydrates per day, depending on the weight and height of a person).

Meal options in regular diets

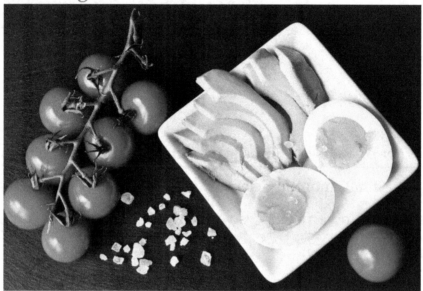

To conquer the weight reduction fight, it becomes tough to continue the dieting combat for a long period. Many people revert to the previous eating patterns after only a few weeks when confronted with the difficulty and limited food ranges of many diets, especially vegan, low-fat and low-calorie diets. For starters, the ketogenic diet is incredibly beneficial for weight reduction, but following specific food choices can be overwhelming. Only after three weeks can you begin noticing significant effects; however, the complications and inconvenience of transitioning to an effective ketogenic diet may deter you from keeping to the program long enough to reap the benefits.

Thankfully, to render your keto diet ever more efficient, successful and simple to use, you will build an array of foods, preparing strategies, tips and suggestions. One hidden tool can be used from the diet's outset, without much details of the keto diet, which is continued even after achieving the weight loss target.

That hidden preferred weapon is the "Fat Bomb."

The Fat Bomb

The fat bombs in the keto diet play a major role in motivation for the dieters. Indulging in a high fat dessert gives you a stress-free environment to continue your diet. These fat bombs provide the correct amounts of fat, carbohydrates, and protein resulting in weight reduction while supplying the user with sustained energy. They do this by supplementing your diet with chemicals that hold your body in a fat-burning state, even after you have had a fulfilling meal.

The Keto diet aims to rely on foods that are high in fat and low in carbs. By modifying what the body utilizes as food, it helps facilitate weight reduction. Carbohydrates, like those present in sugars and bread, are usually transformed into energy. If the body cannot have enough nutrients, the body begins to burn fat as a substitute for energy.

Your liver converts the fat into ketones, which are a form of acid. Getting a certain amount of ketones in your body will lead you to a biochemical condition known as ketosis. Your body can burn stored fat for fuel; thus, you will losing weight when you go through ketosis.

To reach a ketosis condition, it takes between one to ten days of consuming a low-carb, high-fat diet; to sustain the fat-burning cycle of ketosis, you have to continue consuming the keto diet. Eating fatty foods will help you more easily get into ketosis and sustain it for longer periods.

Fat bombs are 90% fat, making them the ideal keto addition for beginners and lifetime keto adherents. They hold you in a ketosis state and can provide health advantages unlike many other high protein foods; you can snack on fat bombs or have them as dinners or as have as a side dish too. They are simple to produce and are available in a range of varieties, from sweet to savory.

Can Fat Bombs Be Healthy?

Ketogenic fat bombs are fueled by two major ingredients: high-fat dairy and coconut oil. Both of these components have several powerful health advantages. Coconut produces a form of fat known as MCTs (medium-chain triglycerides), which gives the body additional ketones that can be readily consumed and used to sustain ketosis.

There are distinct health advantages of consuming high-fat dairy fat bombs. High-fat dairy products produce fatty acids known as CLA (conjugated linoleic acid), minerals and vitamins. Data indicates that CLA plays a significant role in the body's breakdown of fat and may lower cardiac attack and stroke risk.

Eating high-fat dairy meals prior to bedtime may help burn fat when still sleeping. Fat burned while you sleep the body with an energy that does not need to metabolize stress hormones or depend on sugar.

Keto Diet and Mood

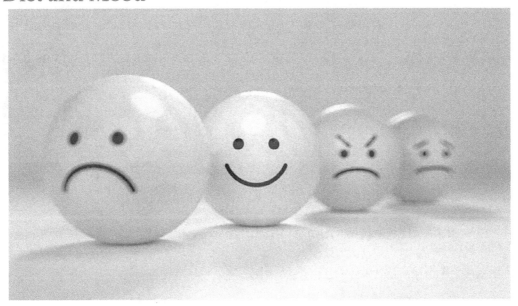

There are various comments from individuals on a keto diet that probably indicate the association between the keto diet and mood changes. Various hypotheses connect the keto diet to mood regulation, even if only partly.

The explanation of why the keto diet aids in accelerated weight reduction and reversal of multiple chronic weight-related problems lead people to come out of the despair of "I am not healthy." As a consequence of the results themselves, most people report a positive attitude by adopting a keto diet. But is that important? What makes a difference is that it has a positive and long-lasting effect. Some research also shows that a ketogenic diet may help combat depression since it provides anti-inflammatory benefits. Inflammations are associated with, at least certain, forms of depression. A few of the advantages are provided below that create the relationship between the keto diet and mood. A keto diet:

1. Helps regulate energy highs and lows.

Ketones offer an immediate energy supply for your brain since they are metabolized quicker than glucose. Ketones give a long-lasting, more accurate and reliable energy supply, and when your body understands it can access your fat reserves for food as well, the brain does not worry.

2. Neurogenesis improvement

Dietary consumption is a crucial element in assessing neurogenesis. A reduced degree of neurogenesis is correlated with multiple depressive illnesses. On the other side, a higher rate increases emotional endurance.

3. Reduces and Brings Down Inflammation

The Keto Diet provides healthy nutritional options, so you avoid consuming inflammatory and refined products. Consuming anti-inflammatory food can have a direct impact on the attitude. If you eat nutritious food high in protein, healthy fats and low-carb vegetables, it reduces inflammation.

4. Feeds the brain.

The good fat you consume on Keto fuels your brain and stabilizes your mood. As your brain is composed of 60% fat, it requires an excess of healthy fats to function properly.

So go ahead and try these easy to make lo carb hi fat desserts and lose weight deliciously!

Chapter 1- Low Carb Desserts

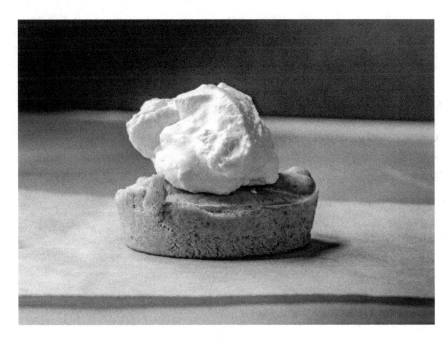

1. 10 Minutes Chocolate Mousse

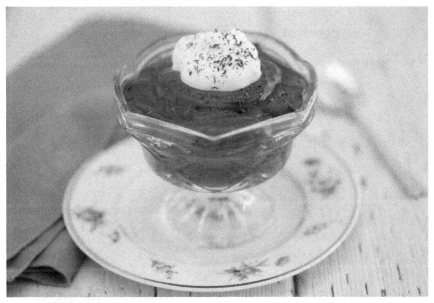

Prep. Time: 10 minutes

Servings: 4

The serving size is ½ cup

Nutrition as per serving:

218 kcal / 23g fat / 5g carbs / 2g fiber / 2g protein = 3g net carbs

Ingredients

- Powdered sweetener 1/4 cup

- Cocoa powder, unsweetened, sifted 1/4 cup

- Vanilla extract 1tsp.

- Heavy whipping cream 1 cup

- Kosher salt 1/4tsp.

Directions

With an electric beater, beat the cream to form stiff peaks. Put in the sweetener, cocoa powder, salt, vanilla and whisk till all ingredients are well combined.

2. The Best Keto Cheesecake

Prep. Time: 20 minutes

Cook Time: 50 minutes

Setting Time: 8 hours

Servings: 12

The serving size is 1 slice

Nutrition as per serving:

600kcal / 54g fat / 7g carbs / 2g fiber / 14g protein = 5 g net carbs

Ingredients

Layer of crust

- Powdered sweetener 1/4 cup

- Almond flour 1 1/2 cups

- Butter melted 6 tbsp.

- Cinnamon 1tsp.

Filling

- Cream cheese, full fat, room temperature (8 oz.)

- Powdered Sweetener 2 Cups

- Eggs at room temperature 5 Large

- Sour cream at room temperature 8 Oz.

- Vanilla extract 1 Tbsp.

Directions

1. Heat the oven to 325F.

2. Arrange the rack in the center of the oven. Mix dry ingredients for the crust in a medium mixing bowl. Mix in the butter. Transfer the crust mixture into a springform pan (10-inch x 4- inch), and using your fingers, press halfway up and around the sides. Then press the mixture with a flat bottom cup into the pan. Chill the crust for about 20 minutes.

3. Beat the cream cheese (at room temperature) in a large mixing container, with an electric beater or a

4. Hand mixer until fluffy and light.

5. If using a stand mixer, attach the paddle accessory.

6. Add in about 1/3rd of sweetener at a time and beat well.

7. Add in one egg at a time beating until well incorporated.

8. Lastly, add in the sour cream, vanilla and mix until just combined.

9. Pour this cheesecake mixture onto the crust and smooth out the top. Place in the heated oven and examine after 50 minutes. The center should not jiggle, and the top should not be glossy anymore.

10. Turn the oven off and open the door slightly, leaving the cheesecake inside for about 30 minutes.

11. Take out the cheesecake and run a knife between the pan and the cheesecake (this is to unstick the cake but don't remove the springform yet). Leave for 1 hour.

12. Chill for at least 8 hrs. loosely covered with plastic wrap.

13. Take off the sides of the springform pan, decorate & serve.

Note: all the ingredients to make the cheesecake should be at room temperature. Anything refrigerated must be left out for at least 4 hrs.

3. Butter Pralines

Prep. Time: 5 minutes

Cook Time: 11 minutes

Chilling Time: 1 hour

Servings: 10

The serving size is 2 Butter Pralines

Nutrition as per serving:

338kcal / 36g fat / 3g carbs / 2g fiber / 2g protein = 1g net carbs

Ingredients

- Salted butter 2 Sticks
- Heavy Cream 2/3 Cup
- Granular Sweetener 2/3 Cup

- Xanthan gum ½ tsp.
- Chopped pecans 2 Cups
- Sea salt

Directions

1. Line parchment paper on a cookie sheet with or apply a silicone baking mat on it.
2. In a saucepan, brown the butter on medium-high heat, stirring regularly, for just about 5 minutes.
3. Add in the sweetener, heavy cream and xanthan gum. Stir and take off the heat.
4. Add in the nuts and chill to firm up, occasionally stirring, for about 1 hour. The mixture will become very thick. Shape into ten cookie forms and place on the lined baking sheet, and sprinkle with the sea salt, if preferred. Let chill until hardened.
5. Keep in a sealed container, keep refrigerated until serving.

4. Homemade Healthy Twix Bars

Prep. Time: 5 minutes

Cook Time: 20 minutes

Servings: 18 Bars

The serving size is 1 Bar

Nutrition as per serving:

111kcal / 7g fat / 8g carbs / 5g fiber / 4g protein = 3g net carbs

Ingredients

For the cookie layer

- Coconut flour 3/4 cup

- Almond flour 1 cup

- Keto maple syrup 1/4 cup

- Sweetener, granulated 1/2 cup

- Flourless keto cookies 1/4 cup

- Almond milk 1/2 cup

For the gooey caramel

- Cashew butter (or any seed or nut butter) 1 cup

- Sticky sweetener of choice 1 cup

- Coconut oil 1 cup

- For the chocolate coating

- Chocolate chips 2 cups

Directions

1. Line parchment paper in a loaf pan or square pan and set aside.

2. In a big mixing bowl, put in almond flour, coconut flour, and then granulated. Combine very well. Mix in the keto syrup and stir to make it into a thick dough.

3. Add the crushed keto cookies and also add a tbsp. of milk to keep it a thick batter. If the batter stays too thick, keep adding milk by tablespoon. Once desired consistency is achieved, shift the batter to the prepared pan and smooth it out. Chill.

4. Combine the cashew butter, coconut oil and syrup on the stovetop or a microwave-safe dish and heat until mixed. Beat very well to make sure the coconut oil is completely mixed. Drizzle the caramel over the prepared cookie layer and shift to the freezer.

5. When the bars are hard, take out of the pan and slice into 18 bars. Once more, put it back in the freezer.

6. Liquefy the chocolate chips by heat. Using two forks, dip each Twix bar into the melted chocolate till evenly covered. Cover all the bars with chocolate. Chill until firm.

5. Best Chocolate Chip cookie

Prep. Time: 5 minutes

Cook Time: 20 minutes

Servings: 15 Cookies

The serving size is 1 Cookie

Nutrition as per serving:

98kcal / 6g fat / 12g carbs / 5g fiber / 5g protein = 7g net carbs

Ingredients

- Almond flour blanched 2 cups
- Baking powder 1 tsp
- Cornstarch 1/4 cup
- Coconut oil 2 tbsp.
- Sticky sweetener, keto-friendly 6 tbsp.
- Almond extract 1 tsp
- Coconut milk, unsweetened 1/4 cup
- Chocolate chips 1/2 cup

Directions

1. Heat oven up to 350F/175C. Line parchment paper on a large cookie tray and put it aside.

2. Place all the dry ingredients in a big mixing bowl, and combine well.

3. Melt the keto-friendly-sticky sweetener, almond extract and coconut oil in a microwave-safe proof or stovetop. Then mix it into the dry mixture, adding milk to combine very well. Stir through your chocolate chips.

4. Form small balls with slightly wet hands from the cookie dough. Set the balls up on the lined cookie tray. Then form them into cookies by pressing them with a fork. Bake for 12 to 15 minutes till they brown.

5. Take out from the oven, allowing to cool on the tray completely.

6. White Chocolate Dairy Free Peanut Butter Cups

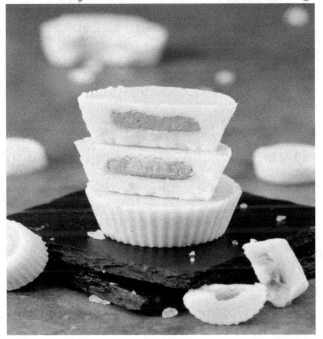

Prep. Time: 5 minutes

Cook Time: 5 minutes

Servings: 40

The serving size is 1 cup

Nutrition as per serving:

117kcal / 6g fat / 14g carbs / 10g fiber / 3g protein = 4g net carbs

Ingredients

- White Chocolate Bar, Sugar-free, coarsely chopped 4 cups

- Peanut butter, smooth (or sunflower seed butter) 1 cup

- Coconut flour 2 tbsp.

- Unsweetened coconut milk 2 tbsp.+ more if needed

Directions

1. Line muffin liners in a standard muffin tin of 12 cups or mini muffin tin of 20 cups and put aside.

2. Removing ½ a cup of your white chocolate, melt the remaining 3 1/2 cups on the stovetop or in a microwave-safe dish, till silky and smooth. Quickly, pour the melted white chocolate equally amongst the prepared muffin cups, scrape down the sides to remove all. Once done, chill

3. Meanwhile, start making the peanut butter filling. Mix the flour and peanut butter well. Adding a tsp. of milk at a time brings to the desired texture.

4. Take the hardened white chocolate cups, then equally pour the peanut butter filling among all of them. After all, is used up, take white chocolate that was kept aside and melt them. Then pour it on each of the cups to cover fully. Chill until firm.

7. Chocolate Crunch Bars

Prep. Time: 5 minutes

Cook Time: 5 minutes

Servings: 20 servings

The serving size is 1 Bar

Nutrition as per serving:

155kcal / 12g fat / 4g carbs / 2g fiber / 7g protein = 2g net carbs

Ingredients

- Chocolate chips (stevia sweetened), 1 1/2 cups
- Almond butter (or any seed or nut butter) 1 cup

- Sticky sweetener (swerve sweetened or monk fruit syrup) 1/2 cup

- Coconut oil 1/4 cup

- Seeds and nuts (like almonds, pepitas, cashews, etc.) 3 cups

Directions

1. Line parchment paper on a baking dish of 8 x 8-inch and put it aside.

2. Combine the keto-friendly chocolate chips, coconut oil, almond butter and sticky sweetener and melt on a stovetop or a microwave-safe dish until combined.

3. Include nuts and seeds and combine until fully mixed. Pour this mixture into the parchment-lined baking dish smoothing it out with a spatula. Chill until firm.

Notes

Keep refrigerated

8. Easy Peanut Butter Cups

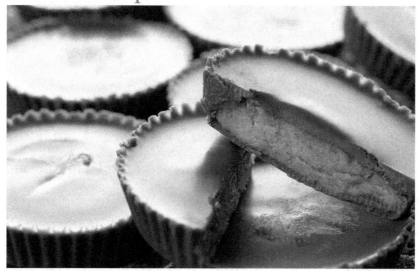

Prep. Time: 10minutes

Cook Time: 5minutes

Servings: 12

The serving size is 1 piece

Nutrition as per serving:

187kcal / 18g fat / 14g carbs / 11g fiber / 3g protein = 3g net carbs

Ingredients

Chocolate layers

- Dark chocolate(not bakers chocolate), Sugar-free, 10 oz. Divided
- Coconut oil 5 tbsp. (divided)
- Vanilla extracts 1/2 tsp. (divided) optional

Peanut butter layer

- Creamy Peanut butter 3 1/2 tbsp.

- Coconut oil 2 tsp.

- Powdered Erythritol (or to taste) 4 tsp.

- Peanut flour 1 1/2 tsp.

- Vanilla extracts 1/8 tsp. Optional

- Sea salt 1 pinch (or to taste) optional

Directions

1. Line parchment liners in a muffin pan

2. Prepare the chocolate layer on the stove, place a double boiler and heat half of the coconut oil and half of the chocolate, stirring regularly, until melted. (Alternatively use a microwave, heat for 20 seconds, stirring at intervals.). Add in half of the vanilla.

3. Fill each lined muffin cup with about 2 tsp. Of chocolate in each. Chill for around 10 minutes till the tops are firm.

4. Prepare the peanut butter filling: in a microwave or a double boiler, heat the coconut oil and peanut butter (similar to step 2). Mix in the peanut flour, powdered sweetener, sea salt and vanilla until smooth. Adjust salt and sweetener to taste if preferred.

5. Pour a tsp. Of the prepared peanut mixture into each cup with the chocolate layer. You don't want it to reach the edges. Chill for 10 minutes more till the tops are firm.

6. Now, prepare a chocolate layer for the top. Heat the leftover coconut oil and chocolate in a microwave or the double boiler (similar to step 2). Add in the vanilla.

7. Pour about 2 tsp of melted chocolate into each cup. It should cover the empty part and the peanut butter circles completely.

8. Again chill for at least 20 to 30 minutes, until completely solid. Keep in the refrigerator.

9. No-Bake Chocolate Coconut Bars

Prep. Time: 1 minute

Cook Time: 5 minutes

Servings: 12 bars

The serving size is 1 bar

Nutrition as per serving:

169 kcal / 17g fat / 5g carbs / 4g fiber / 2g protein = 1g net carbs

Ingredients

- Keto maple syrup 1/4 cup
- Coconut unsweetened, shredded 3 cups
- Coconut oil, melted 1 cup
- Lily's chocolate chips 1-2 cups

Directions

1. Line parchment paper in a large loaf pan or square pan and put aside.
2. Add all the ingredients to a large bowl and combine very well. Shift mixture to the prepared pan. Wet your hands lightly and press them into place. Chill for 30 minutes until firm. Cut into 12 bars.
3. Melt the sugar-free chocolate chips, and using two forks, dip each chilled bar into the melted chocolate and coat evenly. Evenly coat all the bars in the same way. Chill until chocolate solidifies.

4. Keep the Bars in a sealed container at room temperature. If you refrigerated or freeze them, thaw them completely before enjoying them.

10. Chocolate Peanut Butter Hearts

Prep. Time: 5 minutes

Cook Time: 5 minutes

Servings: 20 Hearts

The serving size is 1 Heart

Nutrition as per serving:

95kcal / 6g fat / 7g carbs / 5g fiber / 5g protein = 2g net carbs

Ingredients

• Smooth peanut butter 2 cups

• Sticky sweetener 3/4 cup

• Coconut flour 1 cup

• Chocolate chips of choice 1-2 cups

Directions

1. Line parchment paper on a large tray and put it aside.

2. Combine the keto-friendly sticky sweetener and peanut butter and melt on a stovetop or microwave-safe bowl until combined.

3. Include coconut flour and combine well. If the mixture is too thin, include more coconut flour. Leave for around 10 minutes to thicken.

4. Shape the peanut butter mixture into 18 to 20 small balls. Press each ball in. Then, using a heart-molded cookie cutter, shape the balls into hearts removing excess

peanut butter mixture from the sides. Assemble the hearts on the lined tray and chill.

5. Melt the keto-friendly chocolate chips. With two forks, coat the chocolate by dipping each heart into it. Repeat with all hearts. When done, chill until firm.

Notes

Keep in a sealed jar at room temperature for up to 2 weeks, or refrigerate for up to 2 months.

11. Magic Cookies

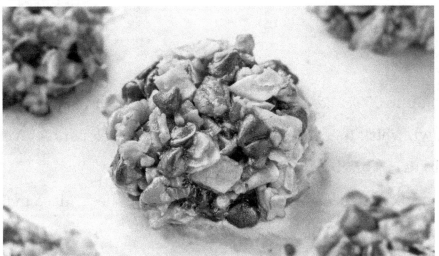

Prep. Time: 10 minutes

Cook Time: 15 minutes

Servings: 15 cookies

The serving size is 1 cookie

Nutrition as per serving:

130kcal / 13g fat / 2g carbs / 1g fiber / 2g protein = 1g net carbs

Ingredients

- Butter softened 3 tbsp.
- Coconut oil 1/4 cup
- Granulated swerve sweetener 3 tbsp.
- Dark chocolate chips, sugar-free (like lily's) 1 cup
- Egg yolks 4 large
- Coconut flakes 1 cup

- Kosher salt 1/2 tsp.

- Walnuts roughly chopped 3/4 cup.

Directions

1. Heat oven up to 350° and line a parchment paper on a baking sheet. In a large mixing bowl, whisk together butter, coconut oil, sweetener, egg yolks and salt; stir in walnuts, coconut, and chocolate chips.

2. Drop spoonfuls of batter onto the prepared baking sheet. Place in the oven and bake for 15 mins until golden,

12. No-Bake Coconut Crack Bars

Prep. Time: 2 minutes

Cook Time: 3 minutes

Servings: 20

The serving size is 1 square

Nutrition as per serving:

108kcal / 11g fat / 2g carbs / 2g fiber /2g protein = 0g net carbs

Ingredients

- Coconut flakes unsweetened & Shredded 3 cups

- Coconut oil, melted 1 cup

- Maple syrup, monk fruit sweetened 1/4 cup (or any liquid sweetener of preference)

Directions

1. Line parchment paper on an 8 x 10-inch pan or an 8 x 8-inch pan and put aside. Or use a loaf pan.

2. Combine unsweetened shredded coconut, melted coconut oil, maple syrup (monk fruit sweetened) in a big mixing bowl and mix till you get a thick batter. If you find it crumbling, add a tsp. of water or a bit of extra syrup.

3. Transfer the coconut mixture to the lined pan. Press firmly with slightly wet hands into place. Chill until firmed. Cut into bars & enjoy!

13. Candied Pecans

Prep. Time: 5 minutes

Cook Time: 1 minute

Servings: 16 Servings

The serving size is 1 Serving

Nutrition as per serving:

139kcal / 15g fat / 3g carbs / 2g fiber / 2g protein = 1g net carbs

Ingredients

- Granulated sweetener divided 1 1/2 cups

- Vanilla extract 1 tsp

- Water 1/4 cup

- Cinnamon 1 tbsp.

- Raw pecans 3 cups

Directions

1. Over medium flame, heat a skillet or large pan.

2. Add 1 cup of the granulated sweetener, vanilla extract and water, and stir until fully mixed. Let it heat up, stirring in between.

3. Once the sweetener is fully melted, include your pecans. Stir around the pecans ensuring every nut is equally coated in the liquid mixture. Keep occasionally stirring till the sweetener starts to set on the pecans. Take off from the heat. Leave for 2 to 3 minutes.

4. Brea apart the pecans with a wooden spoon before they set together.

5. When cooled, mix with the granulated sweetener that was reserved earlier and cinnamon. Store in a sealed container.

14. Sugar-Free Flourless Cookies

Prep. Time: 2 minutes

Cook Time: 10 minutes

Servings: 14 cookies

The serving size is 1 Cookie

Nutrition as per serving:

101kcal / 9g fat / 3g carbs / 1g fiber / 5g protein = 3g net carbs

Ingredients

For the original style:

• Almond butter 1 cup

• Egg 1 large

• Granulated sweetener, stevia blend monk fruit, 3 /4 cup

For the egg-free style:

- Almond butter smooth 1 cup

- Chia seeds, ground 3-4 tbsp.

- Granulated sweetener, stevia blend monk fruit 3/4 cup

Directions

1. Heat the oven up to 350 degrees. Place parchment paper on a cookie sheet or a baking tray.

2. In a big mixing bowl, add all the ingredients and blend until well combined. When using the egg-free recipe, begin with 3 tbsps. of grounded chia seeds. Add an extra tbsp. if the mixture is still too thin.

3. Using your hands or a cookie scoop, shape small balls and place them 3 to 4 inches apart on the baking tray. Make into cookie shape by pressing down with a fork. Bake until cookies are beginning to get a golden brown color but still soft, or for 8 to 10 minutes. Take out from the oven, allowing to cool until firm but soft and chewy.

15. Salted Caramel Fudge

Prep. Time: 5 minutes

Cook Time: 5 minutes

Servings: 24 servings

The serving size is 1 fudge cup

Nutrition as per serving:

148kcal / 15g fat / 4g carbs / 2g fiber / 4g protein = 2g net carbs

Ingredients

- Cashew butter 2 cups
- Keto maple syrup 1/4 cup
- Coconut oil 1/2 cup

Directions

1. Line muffin liners in a mini muffin tin of 24-count and put aside.
2. Combine all the ingredients on a stovetop or in a microwave-safe dish and heat till melted.
3. Take off from heat and beat very well till a glossy, smooth texture remains.
4. Split the fudge mixture equally in the lined muffin tin. Chill for about 30 minutes, till firm.

16. Healthy Kit Kat Bars

Prep. Time: 5 minutes

Cook Time: 5 minutes

Servings: 20 Bars

The serving size is 1 Bar

Nutrition as per serving:

149kcal / 12g fat / 4g carbs / 2g fiber / 7g protein = 2g net carbs

Ingredients

- Keto granola 2 cups
- Almond butter (or any seed or nut butter) 1 cup
- Mixed seeds 1/2 cup
- Coconut oil 1/4 cup
- Mixed nuts 1/2 cup
- Dark chocolate chips, 1 1/2 cups
- Sticky sweetener 1/2 cup

Directions

1. Mix the mixed nuts, keto granola, and seeds in a big bowl. Put aside.
2. Melt the keto chocolate chips on the stovetop or in a microwave-safe dish. Include almond butter, coconut oil, and sticky sweetener. Heat until well combined.
3. Add the melted chocolate mixture onto the dry and combine until fully unified.
4. Shift the kit kat mixture to a pan of 10 x 10-inch lined with parchment. With a spatula, smooth out to a uniform layer. Chill for about 30 minutes, then slice into bars.

Notes: keep refrigerated

17. Healthy No-Bake Keto Cookie Bars

Prep. Time: 5 minutes

Cook Time: 25 minutes

Servings: 12 servings

The serving size is 1 Bar

Nutrition as per serving:

149kcal / 5g fat / 10g carbs / 6g fiber / 10g protein = 4g net carbs

Ingredients

For the cookie

- Almond flour blanched 1 1/2 cups

- Coconut flour 1/4 cup

- Cinnamon, a pinch

- Protein powder, vanilla flavor (optional) 2 scoops

- Granulated sweetener (like

- Sticky sweetener, keto-friendly, 1/2 cup

- Monk fruit sweetener) 2 tbsp.

- Vanilla extract 1/2 tsp

- Cashew butter (or any nut butter) 1/2 cup

- Sticky sweetener, keto-friendly, 1/2 cup

- Almond milk 1 tbsp.

For the protein icing

- Protein powder,

- Vanilla flavor 3 scoops

- Granulated sweetener, keto-friendly 1-2 tbsp. + for sprinkling 1/2 tsp

- Almond milk, (for batter) 1 tbsp.

For the coconut butter icing

- Coconut butter melted 4-6 tbsp.

- Sticky sweetener, 2 tbsp.

- Almond milk 1 tbsp.

Directions

1. Preparing sugar cookie base

2. Place tin foil in a baking pan of 8 x 8 inches and put aside.

3. Mix the protein powder, flours, granulated sweetener and cinnamon in a big mixing bowl, and put aside.

4. Melt the sticky sweetener with cashew butter on a stovetop or a microwave-proof bowl. Stir in the vanilla extract and add to the dry mixture. Beat superbly until fully combined. If the batter formed is too thick, add a tablespoon of almond milk with a tablespoon and mix well until desired consistency.

5. Pour the batter into the lined baking sheet and press tightly in place. Scatter the ½ teaspoon of keto-friendly granulated sweetener and chill for about 15 minutes until they are firm. Then add an icing of choice and chill for 30 minutes more to settle the icing before slicing.

6. Preparing the icing(s)

7. Mix all ingredients of the icings (separately) and, using almond milk, thin down the mixture till a very thick icing is formed.

18. Keto Chocolate Bark with Almonds and Bacon

Prep. Time: 30 minutes

Servings: 8 servings

The serving size is 1/8 of the recipe

Nutrition as per serving:

157kcal /12.8g fat / 4g protein / 7.5g fiber / 12.7g carbs = 5.2g net carbs

Ingredients

- Sugar-free Chocolate Chips 1 bag (9 oz.)
- Chopped Almonds 1/2 cup
- Bacon cooked & crumbled2 slices

Directions

1. In a microwave-safe bowl, melt the chocolate chips on high in 30 seconds intervals, stirring every time until all chocolate is melted.
2. Include the chopped almonds into the melted chocolate and mix.
3. Line a baking sheet with parchment and pour the chocolate mixture on it in a thin layer of about 1/2 inch.
4. Immediately top the chocolate with the crumbled bacon and press in with a flat spoon.
5. Chill for around 20 minutes or till the chocolate has solidified. Peel the parchment away from the hardened chocolate and crack it into eight pieces. Keep refrigerated.

Chapter 2- Chaffles

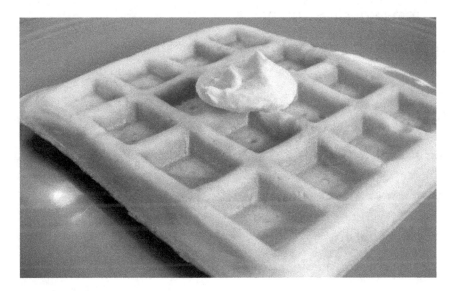

1. Basic chaffle recipe

Prep. Time: 5 minutes

Cook Time: 5 minutes

Servings: 1 chaffle

The serving size is 1 chaffle

Nutrition as per serving:

291kcal / 23g fat / 1g carbs / 0g fiber / 20g protein = 1g net carbs

Ingredients

- Sharp cheddar cheese shredded 1/2 cup

- Eggs 1

Directions

1. Whisk the egg.

2. In the waffle maker, assemble 1/4 cup of shredded cheese.

3. Top the cheese with beaten egg.

4. Top with the remainder 1/4 cup of cheese.

5. Cook till it's golden and crispy. It will get crispier as it cools.

2. Keto Oreo Chaffles

Prep. Time: 15 minutes

Cook Time: 8 minutes

Servings: 2 full-size chaffles or 4 mini chaffles

The serving size is 2 chaffles

Nutrition as per serving:

381kcal / 14.6g fat / 14g carbs / 5g fiber / 17g protein = 9g net carbs

Ingredients

- Sugar-Free Chocolate Chips 1/2 cup

- Butter 1/2 cup

- Eggs 3

- Truvia 1/4 cup

- Vanilla extract 1tsp.

- For Cream Cheese Frosting

- Butter, room temperature 4 oz.

- Cream Cheese, room temperature 4 oz.

- Powdered Swerve 1/2 cup

- Heavy Whipping Cream 1/4 cup

- Vanilla extract 1tsp.

Directions

1. Melt the butter and chocolate for around 1 minute in a microwave-proof dish. Stir well. You really ought to use the warmth within the chocolate and butter to melt most of the clumps. You have overheated the chocolate; when you microwave, and all is melted, it means you have overheated the chocolate. So grab yourself a spoon and begin stirring. If required, add 10 seconds, but stir just before you plan to do so.

2. Put the eggs, vanilla and sweetener, in a bowl and whisk until fluffy and light.

3. In a steady stream, add the melted chocolate into the egg mix and whisk again until well-combined.

4. In a Waffle Maker, pour around 1/4 of the mixture and cook for 7 to-8 minutes until it's crispy.

5. Prepare the frosting as they are cooking.

6. Put all the frosting ingredients into a food processor bowl and mix until fluffy and smooth. To achieve the right consistency, include a little extra cream.

7. To create your Oreo Chaffle, spread or pipe the frosting evenly in between the two chaffles.

8. The waffle machine, do not overfill it! It will create a giant mess and ruin the batter and the maker, utilizing no more than 1/4 cup of the batter.

9. Leave the waffles to cool down a bit before frosting. It is going to help them to remain crisp.

10. To make the frosting, use room-temp butter and cream cheese.

3. Glazed Donut Chaffle

Prep. Time: 10 mins

Cook Time: 5 mins

Servings: 3 chaffles

The serving size is 1 chaffle

Nutrition as per serving:

312kcal / 15g fat / 6g carbs / 1g fiber / 9g protein = 5g net carbs

Ingredients

For the chaffles

- Mozzarella cheese shredded ½ cup

- Whey protein isolates Unflavored 2 tbsp.

- Cream Cheese 1 oz.

- Swerve confectioners (Sugar substitute) 2 tbsp.

- Vanilla extract ½tsp.

- Egg 1

- Baking powder ½tsp.

For the glaze topping:

- Heavy whipping cream2 tbsp.

- Swerve confectioners (sugar substitute) 3-4 tbsp.

- Vanilla extract ½tsp.

Directions

1. Turn on the waffle maker.

2. In a microwave-proof bowl, combine the cream cheese and mozzarella cheese. Microwave at 30-second breaks until it is all melted and stir to combine completely.

3. Include the whey protein, baking powder, 2 tbsp. Keto sweetener to the melted cheese, and work with your hands to knead until well combined.

4. Put the dough in a mixing bowl, and whisk in the vanilla and egg into it to form a smooth batter.

5. Put 1/3 of the mixture into the waffle machine, and let it cook for 3 to 5 minutes.

6. Repeat the above step 5 to make a total of three chaffles.

7. Whisk the glaze topping ingredients together and drizzle on top of the chaffles generously before serving.

4. Keto Pumpkin Chaffles

Prep. Time: 2 mins

Cook Time: 5 mins

Servings: 2 chaffles

The serving size is 2 chaffles

Nutrition as per serving: (without toppings)

250kcal / 15g fat / 5g carbs / 1g fiber / 23g protein = 4g net carbs

Ingredients

- Mozzarella cheese, shredded ½ cup

- Egg, beaten 1 whole

- Pumpkin purée 1 ½ tbsp.

- Swerve confectioners ½tsp.

- Vanilla extract ½tsp.

- Pumpkin pie spice ¼tsp.

- Pure maple extract ⅛tsp.

- For topping- optional

- roasted pecans, cinnamon, whip cream and sugar-free maple syrup

Directions

1. Switch on the Waffle Maker and begin preparing the mixture.

2. Add all the given ingredients to a bowl, except for the mozzarella cheese, and whisk. Include the cheese and combine until well mixed.

3. Grease the waffle plates and put half the mixture into the middle of the plate. Cover the lid for 4- to 6 minutes, based on how crispy Chaffles you like.

4. Take it out and cook the second one. Serve with all or some mix of toppings, like sugar-free maple syrup, butter, roasted pecans, and a dollop of whipping cream or ground cinnamon dust.

5. Cream Cheese Chaffle with Lemon Curd

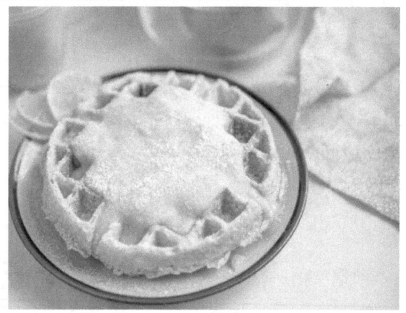

Prep. Time: 5 minutes

Cook Time: 4 minutes

Additional Time: 40 minute

Servings: 2-3 serving

The serving size is 1 chaffle

Nutrition as per serving:

302 kcals / 24g fat / 6g carbs / 1g fiber / 15g protein = 5g net carbs

Ingredients

- One batch keto lemon curd (recipe here)
- Eggs 3 large
- Cream cheese softened 4 oz.
- Lakanto monkfruit (or any low carb sweetener) 1 tbsp.

- Vanilla extract 1tsp.

- Mozzarella cheese shredded 3/4 cup

- Coconut flour 3 tbsp.

- Baking powder 1tsp.

- Salt 1/3tsp.

- Homemade keto whipped cream (optional) (recipe here)

Directions

1. Prepare lemon curd according to Directions and let cool in the refrigerator.

2. Turn on the waffle maker and grease it with oil.

3. Take a small bowl, put coconut flour, salt and baking powder. Combine and put aside.

4. Take a large bowl, put cream cheese, eggs, vanilla and sweetener. With an electric beater, beat until foamy. You may see chunks of cream cheese, and that is okay.

5. Include mozzarella cheese into the egg mixture and keep beating.

6. Pour the dry ingredients into the egg mixture and keep mixing until well blended.

7. Put batter into the preheated waffle machine and cook.

8. Take off from waffle machine; spread cooled lemon curd, top with keto whipped cream and enjoy.

6. Strawberries & Cream Keto Chaffles

Prep. Time: 25 minutes

Cook Time: 10 minutes

Servings: 8 chaffles

The serving size is 1 chaffle

Nutrition as per serving:

328cals / 12g fat / 8g carbs / 4g fiber /6g protein = 4g net carbs

Ingredients

- Cream cheese 3 oz.
- Mozzarella cheese, shredded 2 cups
- Eggs, beaten 2
- Almond flour 1/2 cup
- Swerve confectioner sweetener 3 tbsp. + 1 tbsp.
- Baking powder 2tsps
- Strawberries 8
- Whipped cream 1 cup (canister - 2 tbsp. Per waffle)

Directions

1. In a microwavable dish, add the mozzarella and cream cheese, cook for 1 minute, mixing well. If the cheese is all melted, then go to the next step. Else cook for another 30 seconds stirring well.
2. Take another bowl, whisk eggs, including the almond flour, 3 tbsp. of keto sweetener, and baking powder.
3. Include the melted cheese mixture into the egg and almond flour mixture and combine well. Carefully add in 2 strawberries coarsely chopped. Chill for 20 minutes.
4. Meanwhile, slice the unused strawberries and mix with 1 tbsp. of Swerve. Chill.
5. Take out the batter from the refrigerator after 20 minutes. Heat the waffle iron and grease it.

6. Put 1/4 cup of the batter in the mid of the heated waffle iron. Ensuring the waffles are small makes it easier to remove from the waffle maker.

7. Transfer to a plate when cooked and cool before adding whipped cream and topping with strawberries.

This recipe gave me eight small waffles.

7. Keto Peanut Butter Cup Chaffle

Prep. Time: 2 minutes

Cook Time: 5 minutes

Servings: 2 Chaffles

The serving size is 1 chaffle + filling

Nutrition as per serving:

264kcal / 21.6g fat / 7.2g carbs / 2g fiber / 9.45g protein = 4.2g net carbs

Ingredients

For the Chaffle

- Heavy Cream 1 tbsp.

- Vanilla Extract 1/2 tsp

- Egg 1

- Cake Batter Flavor 1/2 tsp

- Unsweetened Cocoa 1 tbsp.

- Coconut Flour 1 tsp

- Lakanto Powdered Sweetener 1 tbsp.

- Baking Powder 1/4 tsp

For Peanut Butter Filling

- Heavy Cream 2 tbsp.

- All-natural Peanut Butter 3 tbsp.

- Lakanto Powdered Sweetener 2 tsp

Directions

1. Preheat a waffle maker.

2. Combine all the chaffle ingredients in a small mixing bowl.

3. Put half of the chaffle batter into the middle of the waffle machine and cook for 3 to 5 minutes.

4. Cautiously remove and duplicate for the second chaffle. Leave chaffles for a couple of minutes to let them crisp up.

5. Prepare the peanut butter filling by blending all the ingredients together and layer between chaffles.

8. Vanilla Chocolate Chip

Prep. Time: 1 minute

Cook Time: 4 minutes

Servings: 1 serving

The serving size is 1 large or 2 mini chaffle

Nutrition as per serving:

297.6 kcal. / 20.1g fat / 5.2g carbs / 1.5g fiber / 22.2g protein = 3.9g net carbs

Ingredients

- Mozzarella shredded 1/2 cup

- Eggs 1 medium
- Granulated sweetener keto 1 tbsp.
- Vanilla extract 1 tsp
- Almond meal or flour 2 tbsp.
- Chocolate chips, sugar-free 1 tbsp.

Directions

1. Mix all the ingredients in a large bowl.
2. Turn on the waffle maker. When it is heated, grease with olive oil and put half the mixture into the waffle machine. Cook for 2 to 4 minutes, then take out and repeat. It will make 2 small-chaffles per recipe.
3. Enjoy with your favorite toppings.

9. Chaffle Churro

Prep. Time: 10 minutes

Cook Time: 6-10 minutes

Servings: 2

The serving size is 4 churros

Nutrition as per serving:

189 kcals / 14.3g fat / 5.g carbs / 1g fiber / 10g protein = 4g net carbs

Ingredients

- Egg 1
- Almond flour 1 Tbsp.
- Vanilla extract ½ tsp.
- Cinnamon divided 1 tsp.

- Baking powder ¼ tsp.

- Shredded mozzarella ½ cup.

- Swerve confectioners (or any sugar substitute) 1 Tbsp.

- Swerve brown sugar (keto-friendly sugar substitute) 1 Tbsp.

- Butter melted 1 Tbsp.

Directions

1. Heat the waffle iron.

2. Combine the almond flour, egg, vanilla extract, baking powder, ½ tsp of cinnamon, swerve confectioners' sugar and shredded mozzarella in a bowl, and stir to combine well.

3. Spread half of the batter equally onto the waffle iron, and let it cook for 3 to 5 minutes. Cooking for more time will give a crispier chaffle.

4. Take out the cooked chaffle and pour the remaining batter onto it. Close the lid and cook for about 3 to 5 minutes.

5. Make both the chaffles into strips.

6. Put the cut strips in a bowl and drizzle on melted butter generously.

7. In another bowl, stir together the keto brown sugar and the leftover ½ tsp of cinnamon until well-combined.

8. Toss the churro chaffle strips in the sugar-cinnamon mixture in the bowl to coat them evenly.

10. Keto Cauliflower Chaffles Recipe

Prep. Time: 5 minutes

Cook Time: 4 minutes

Servings: 2 chaffles

The serving size is 2 chaffles

Nutrition as per serving:

246kcal / 16g fat / 7g carbs / 2g fiber / 20g protein = 5g net carbs

Ingredients

- Riced cauliflower 1 cup
- Garlic powder 1/4tsp.
- Ground black pepper 1/4tsp.
- Italian seasoning 1/2tsp.
- Kosher salt 1/4tsp.
- Mozzarella cheese shredded 1/2 cup
- Eggs 1
- Parmesan cheese shredded 1/2 cup

Directions

1. In a blender, add all the ingredients and blend well. Turn the waffle maker on.
2. Put 1/8 cup of parmesan cheese onto the waffle machine. Ensure to cover up the bottom of the waffle machine entirely.
3. Cover the cheese with the cauliflower batter, then sprinkle another layer of parmesan cheese on the cauliflower mixture. Cover and cook.
4. Cook for 4 to 5 minutes, or till crispy.
5. Will make 2 regular-size chaffles or 4 mini chaffles.
6. It freezes well. Prepare a big lot and freeze for the future.

11. Zucchini Chaffles

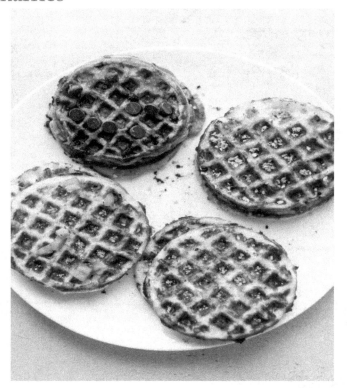

Prep. Time: 10 minutes

Cook Time: 5 minutes

Servings: 2 chaffles

The serving size is 1 chaffle

Nutrition as per serving:

194kcal / 13g fat / 4g carbs / 1g fiber / 16g protein = 3g net carbs

Ingredients

• Zucchini, grated 1 cup

• Eggs, beaten 1

• Parmesan cheese shredded 1/2 cup

- Mozzarella cheese shredded 1/4 cup

- Dried basil, 1tsp. Or fresh basil, chopped 1/4 cup

- Kosher Salt, divided 3/4tsp.

- Ground Black Pepper 1/2tsp.

Directions

1. Put the shredded zucchini in a bowl and Sprinkle salt, about 1/4tsp on it and leave it aside to gather other ingredients. Moments before using put the zucchini in a paper towel, wrap and press to wring out all the extra water.

2. Take a bowl and whisk in the egg. Include the mozzarella, grated zucchini, basil, and pepper 1/2tsp of salt.

3. Cover the waffle maker base with a layer of 1 to 2 tbsp. of the shredded parmesan.

4. Then spread 1/4 of the zucchini batter. Spread another layer of 1 to 2 tbsp. of shredded parmesan and shut the lid.

5. Let it cook for 4 to 8 minutes. It depends on the dimensions of your waffle machine. Normally, once the chaffle is not emitting vapors of steam, it is nearly done. For the greatest results, let it cook until good and browned.

6. Take out and duplicate for the next waffle.

Will make 4 small chaffles or 2 full-size chaffles in a Mini waffle maker.

12. Keto Pizza Chaffle

Prep. Time: 10 minutes

Cook Time: 30 minutes

Servings: 2 servings

The serving size is 1 chaffle

Nutrition as per serving:

76 kcal / 4.3g fat / 4.1g carbs / 1.2g fiber / 5.5g protein = 3.2g net carbs

Ingredients

- Egg 1

- Mozzarella cheese shredded 1/2 cup

- Italian seasoning a pinch

- Pizza sauce No sugar added 1 tbsp.

- Toppings – pepperoni, shredded cheese (or any other toppings)

Directions

- Heat the waffle maker.

- Whisk the egg, and Italian seasonings in a small mixing bowl, together.

- Stir in the cheese, leaving a few tsps. for layering.

- Layer a tsp of grated cheese onto the preheated waffle machine and allow it to cook for about 30 seconds.

- It will make a crispier crust.

- Pour half the pizza mixture into the waffle maker and allow to cook for around 4 minutes till it's slightly crispy and golden brown!

- Take out the waffle and make the second chaffle with the remaining mixture.

- Spread the pizza sauce, pepperoni and shredded cheese. Place in Microwave and heat on high for around 20 seconds and done! On the spot Chaffle PIZZA!

13. Crispy Taco Chaffle Shells

Prep. Time: 5 minutes

Cook Time: 8 minutes

Servings: 2 chaffles

The serving size is 1 chaffle

Nutrition as per serving:

258kcal / 19g fat / 4g carbs / 2g fiber / 18g protein = 2g net carbs

Ingredients

- Egg white 1
- Monterey jack cheese shredded 1/4 cup
- Sharp cheddar cheese shredded 1/4 cup
- Water 3/4 tsp
- Coconut flour 1 tsp
- Baking powder 1/4 tsp
- Chili powder 1/8 tsp
- Salt a pinch

Directions

1. Turn on the Waffle iron and lightly grease it with oil when it is hot.

2. In a mixing bowl, mix all of the above ingredients and blend to combine.

3. Pour half of the mixture onto the waffle iron and shut the lid. Cook for 4 minutes without lifting the lid. The chaffle will not set in less than 4 minutes.

4. Take out the cooked taco chaffle and put it aside. Do the same process with the remaining chaffle batter.

5. Put a muffin pan upside down and assemble the taco chaffle upon the cups to make into a taco shell. Put aside for a few minutes.

6. When it is firm, fill it with your favorite Taco Meat fillings. Serve.

Enjoy this delicious keto crispy taco chaffle shell with your favorite toppings.

Chapter 3- Keto Cakes and Cupcakes

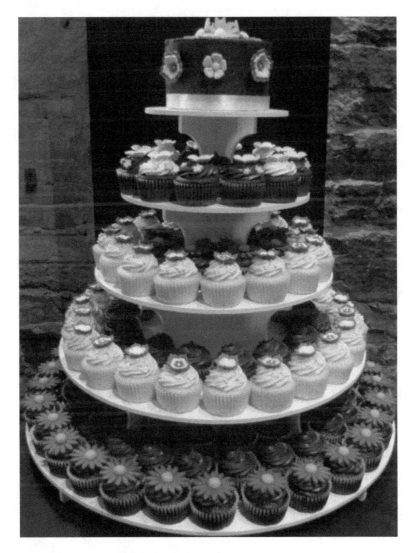

1. Chocolate Cake with Chocolate Icing

Prep. Time: 10 minutes

Cook Time: 25 minutes

Servings: 9 slices

The serving size is 1 slice

Nutrition as per serving:

358kcal / 33g fat / 11g carbs / 6g fiber / 8g protein = 5g net carbs

Ingredients

- Coconut flour 3/4 cup
- Granular sweetener 3/4 cup
- Cocoa powder 1/2 cup
- Baking powder 2tsps
- Eggs 6
- Heavy whipping cream 2/3 cup
- Melted butter 1/2 cup
- For chocolate icing
- Heavy whipping cream 1 cup
- Keto granular sweetener 1/4 cup
- Vanilla extracts 1tsp.
- Cocoa powder sifted 1/3 cup

Directions

1. Heat the oven up to 350F.
2. Oil a cake pan of 8x8.
3. In a large mixing bowl, put all the cake ingredients to blend well with an electric mixer or a stand mixer.
4. Transfer the batter to the oiled pan and put in the heated oven for 25 minutes or till a toothpick inserted in the center comes out clean.
5. Take out from the oven. Leave to cool fully before icing.
6. Prepare the Icing

7. With an electric mixer, beat the whipping cream until stiff peaks form. Include the cocoa powder, swerve, and vanilla. Keep beating until just combined.

8. Spread the icing evenly all over the cake and serve. Keep any remains in the refrigerator.

2. 4 Ingredients Cheesecake Fluff

Prep. Time: 10 minutes

Servings: 6

The serving size is ½ cup

Nutrition as per serving:

258kcal / 27g fat / 4g carbs / 0g fiber / 4g protein = 4g net carbs

Ingredients

- Heavy Whipping Cream1 Cup

- Cream Cheese, Softened 1 Brick (8 oz.)

- Lemon Zest 1 tsp.

- Keto-friendly Granular Sweetener 1/2 Cup

Directions

1. Prepare the Fluff

2. Put the heavy cream in a bowl of a stand mixer and beat until stiff peaks begin to form. An electric beater or a hand beater can also be used.

3. Transfer the whipped cream into a separate bowl and put aside

4. To the same stand mixer bowl, add the cream cheese (softened), sweetener, zest, and whisk until smooth.

5. Now add the whipped cream to the cream cheese into the mixer bowl. Fold with a spatula gently till it is halfway combined. Finish whipping with the stand mixer until smooth.

6. Top with your fave toppings and serve.

3. Mug Cake Peanut Butter, Chocolate or Vanilla

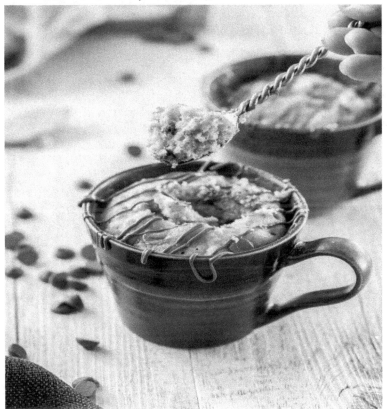

Prep. Time: 4 minutes

Cook Time: 1 minute

Servings: 1

The serving size is 1 mug cake

Nutrition as per serving:

(For mug cake with almond flour: chocolate flavor and no chocolate chips)

312 kcal / 7 carbs/ 28g fat / 12g protein/4g fiber = 3 net carbs

(Peanut butter flavor and no chocolate chips)

395 kcal / 8 carbs /35g fat / 15g protein/4g fiber = 5 net carb

(Vanilla flavor and no chocolate chips)

303 kcal / 5 carbs/ 28g fat / 11g protein /2g fiber = 3 net carb

Ingredients

- Butter melted 1 Tbsp.
- Almond flour 3 Tbsp. or Coconut flour 1 Tbsp.
- Granular Sweetener 2 Tbsp.
- Sugar-free Peanut butter 1 Tbsp. (For Peanut Butter flavor)
- Cocoa powder 1 Tbsp. (For Chocolate flavor)
- Baking powder ½ tsp.
- Egg, beaten 1
- Sugar-free Chocolate Chips 1 Tbsp.
- Vanilla few drops

Directions

For Vanilla flavor

1. In a microwave-proof coffee mug, heat the butter for 10 seconds to melt in the microwave.
2. Include the almond flour or coconut flour, baking powder, sweetener, beaten egg and vanilla. Combine well.
3. For 60 seconds, microwave on high, ensuring not to overcook; otherwise, it will come out dry. Sprinkle keto chocolate chips on top if preferred or stir in before cooking.

For Chocolate flavor

In a microwave-proof coffee mug, heat the butter for 10 seconds to melt in the microwave. Include the almond flour or coconut flour, cocoa powder, sweetener, baking powder, beaten egg and vanilla. Combine well. For 60 seconds, microwave on high, ensuring not to overcook; it will come out dry. Sprinkle keto chocolate chips on top if preferred.

For Peanut Butter flavor

1. In a microwave-proof coffee mug, heat the butter for 10 seconds to melt in the microwave.
2. Include the almond flour or coconut flour, baking powder, sweetener, beaten egg and vanilla. Combine well. Stir in peanut butter. For 60 seconds, microwave on high, ensuring not to overcook; otherwise, it will come out dry. Sprinkle keto chocolate chips on top if preferred.

Directions for Baking: Bake in an oven-safe small bowl. Bake in the oven for 15 to 20 minutes at 350.

4. Chocolate Coconut Flour Cupcakes

Prep. Time: 10 minutes

Cook Time: 25 minutes

Servings: 12 cupcakes

The serving size is 1 cupcake

Nutrition as per serving:

268 kcal / 22g fat / 6g carbs / 3g fiber / 6g protein = 3g net carbs

Ingredients

For Cupcakes:

- Butter melted 1/2 cup

- Cocoa powder 7 tbsp.

- Instant coffee granules 1 tsp (optional)

- Eggs at room temperature 7

- Vanilla extracts 1 tsp

- Coconut flour 2/3 cup

- Baking powder 2 tsp

- Swerve sweetener 2/3 cup

- Salt 1/2 tsp

- Hemp milk or unsweetened almond milk 1/2 cup (+more)

For Espresso Buttercream:

- Hot water 2 tbsp.

- Instant coffee or instant espresso powder 2 tsp

- Whipping cream 1/2 cup

- Butter softened 6 tbsp.

- Cream cheese softened 4 oz.

- Swerve powdered sweetener 1/2 cup

Directions

For Cupcakes:

1. Heat the oven up to 350F and line silicone liners or parchment on a muffin tin.

2. Mix together the cocoa powder, melted butter, and espresso powder in a large mixing bowl,

3. Include the vanilla and eggs and whisk until well combined. Now add in the coconut flour, baking powder, salt and sweetener, and mix until smooth.

4. Pour the almond milk in and stir. If the batter is very thick, add in 1 tbsp. of almond milk at a time to thin it out. It should not be pourable but of scoopable consistency.

5. Scoop the batter equally among the prepared muffin tins and put in the oven's center rack, baking for 20-25 minutes. Check the cupcakes with a tester inserted into the center comes out clean, then cupcakes are done. Leave to cool in the pan for 5 to 10 minutes, and then cool completely on a wire rack.

For Buttercream:

1. Dissolve the coffee in hot water. Put aside.

2. Whip cream using an electric mixer until stiff peaks are formed. Put aside.

3. Beat cream cheese, butter, and sweetener all together in a medium mixing bowl until creamy. Include coffee mixture and mix until combined. fold in the whipped cream Using a rubber spatula carefully till well combined.

4. Layer frosting on the cooled cupcakes with an offset spatula or a knife.

5. Low-carb red velvet cupcakes/ cake

Prep. Time: 15-30 minutes

Cook Time: 20-25 minutes

Servings: 12 slice

The serving size is 1 slice

Nutrition as per serving:

193kcals / 12g fat / 6.4g carbs / 1g fiber / 5.9g protein = 5.4g net carbs

Ingredients

- Almond flour 1+ 3/4 cups

- Swerve confectioner sweetener (not substitutes) 2/3 cup

- Cocoa powder 2 tbsp.

- Baking powder 2tsp.

- Baking soda 1/2tsp.

- Eggs 2

- Full fat coconut milk 1/2 cup + 2 tbsp.

- Olive oil 3 tbsp.

- Apple cider vinegar 1 tbsp.

- Vanilla extract 1 tbsp.

- Red food coloring 2 tbsp.

For frosting

- Cream cheese at room temperature 1 container (8 oz.)

- Butter softened 2 ½ tbsp.

- Swerve confectioner sweetener 1 cup

- Coconut milk 2 ½ tbsp.

- Vanilla extract 1tsp.

- Salt 1/8tsp.

**Double Frosting for Layer Cake

Directions

1. Preheat oven to 350 degrees

2. In a large mixing bowl, add the wet ingredients, eggs, milk, vanilla extract, olive oil, apple cider vinegar and food coloring. Blend until smooth.

3. Now sift together the cocoa powder, Swerve Confectioner, baking powder and baking soda, add to the wet ingredients, and incorporate it into the batter with an electric mixer or a hand whisk.

4. Lastly, sift in the almond flour. Moving the flour back and forth with a whisk will speed up the process significantly. Fold the sifted flour gently into the batter till smooth and all is well incorporated. Use the batter immediately.

5. To make Cupcakes: Scoop batter into the muffin liners, fill only up to 2/3 of liner -do not over-fill. Ensure the oven is heated, put in the oven for 15 minutes at 350 degrees, and then turn the muffin tin in 180 degrees and cook for an extra 10 minutes. (Bear in mind, oven times vary occasionally - humidity and altitude can impact things, so watch closely as they may need a few minutes more or even less).

6. Take out from the oven, do not remove from pan and set aside to cool completely.

7. For Layer Cake: 2 Layer- line parchment paper in two cake pans (8 inches each) and oil the sides. Transfer batter to both pans evenly. Use a wet spatula to spread

the batter smoothly. Apply the same process for three layers, but using thinner pans as dividing the batter three ways-every layers will become thin.

8. Place pans into oven for 20-25 minutes baking at 350 degrees. Cautiously turn the pans 180 degrees halfway through baking and cover lightly with a foil. At 20 to 25 minutes, take out the pans; they will be a bit soft. Set them aside to cool completely. When they are cool, take a knife and run it around the side of the pan and turn them over carefully onto a plate or cooling rack and leave them for an extra 5 to 10 minutes before icing.

9. Meanwhile, prepare. Blend the softened butter and cream cheese together With an electric beater. Include milk and vanilla extract and beat again. Lastly, sift in the Swerve, salt mixing well one last time. If you want a thicker frosting, chill it in the refrigerator. Or adding more Swerve will give a thicker texture or add more milk to make it thinner. * For a layer cake, double the frosting recipe.

10. Spread or pipe frosting onto cupcakes, sprinkle some decoration if desired and enjoy!! To frost layer cake, it is simpler to first chill the layers in the freezer. Then frost and pile each layer to end frost the sides and top.

Keep any leftovers in a sealed box and refrigerate. Enjoy!

6. Vanilla Cupcakes

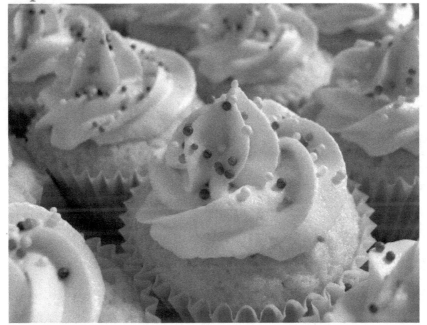

Prep. Time: 5 minutes

Cook Time: 20 minutes

Servings: 10 Cupcakes

The serving size is 1 cupcake

Nutrition as per serving:

153kcal / 13g fat / 4g carbs / 2g fiber / 5g protein = 2g net carbs

Ingredients

- Butter 1/2 cup

- Keto granulated sweetener 2/3 cup

- Vanilla extract 2 tsp

- Eggs whisked * See notes 6 large

- Milk of choice ** See notes 2 tbsp.

- Coconut flour 1/2 cup

- Baking powder 1 tsp

- Keto vanilla frosting 1 batch

Directions

1. Heat the oven up to 350F/180C. Place muffin liners in a 12-cup muffin tin and oil 10 of them.

2. Beat the butter, salt, sugar, eggs and vanilla extract together in a big mixing bowl when combined-well include the milk and mix until blended.

3. In another bowl, sift the baking powder and coconut flour together. Add the wet ingredients to the dry and mix until combined.

4. Pour the batter equally into the ten muffin cups, filling up to ¾ full. Place the cupcakes on the middle rack and bake for 17 to 20 minutes until the muffin top springs back to touch

5. Remove the muffin pan from the oven, set it aside to cool for 10 minutes, and then cool completely on a wire rack. Frost, when cooled.

7. Healthy Flourless Fudge Brownies

Prep. Time: 5 minutes

Cook Time: 20 minutes

Servings: 12 servings

The serving size is 1 Brownie

Nutrition as per serving:

86kcal / 5g fat / 5g carbs / 3g fiber / 7g protein = 2g net carbs

Ingredients

- Pumpkin puree 2 cups

- Almond butter 1 cup

- Cocoa powder 1/2 cup

- Granulated sweetener (or liquid stevia drops) 1/4 cup

For the Chocolate Coconut Frosting

- Chocolate chips 2 cups

- Coconut milk canned 1 cup

- For the chocolate protein frosting

- Protein powder, chocolate flavor 2 scoops

- Granulated sweetener 1-2 tbsp.

- Seed or nut butter of choice 1-2 tbsp.

- Milk or liquid *1 tbsp.

For the Cheese Cream Frosting

- Cream cheese 125 grams

- Cocoa powder 1-2 tbsp.

- Granulated sweetener of choice 1-2 tbsp.

Directions

1. For the fudge brownies

2. Heat the oven up to 350 degrees, oil a loaf pan or small cake pan and put aside.

3. Melt the nut butter in a small microwave-proof bowl. In a big mixing bowl, put in the pumpkin puree, dark cocoa powder, nut butter, and combine very well.

4. Transfer the mixture to the oiled pan and put in preheated oven for around 20 to 25 minutes or until fully baked. Remove from the oven, set aside to cool completely. When cooled, apply the frosting and chill for about 30 minutes to settle.

Preparing the cream cheese or protein frosting:

1. In a big mixing bowl, mix together all the ingredients and beat well. With a tablespoon. keep adding dairy-free milk till a frosting consistency is reached.

2. For the coconut chocolate ganache

3. In a microwave-proof bowl, combine all the ingredients and heat gradually until just mixed- whisk till a glossy and thick frosting remains.

8. Healthy Keto Chocolate Raspberry Mug Cake
Prep. Time: 1 minute

Cook Time: 1 minute

Servings: 1 serving

The serving size is 1 mug cake

Nutrition as per serving:

152kcal / 8g fat / 13g carbs / 8g fiber / 7g protein = 5g net carbs

Ingredients

- Coconut flour 1 tbsp.

- Granulated sweetener of choice 1 tbsp.

- Cocoa powder 2 tbsp.

- Baking powder 1/4 tsp

- Sunflower seed butter (or any seed or nut butter) 1 tbsp.

- Pumpkin puree 3 tbsp.

- Frozen or fresh raspberries 1/4 cup

- Coconut milk unsweetened 1-2 tbsp.

Directions

1. In a microwave-proof mug, put in the dry ingredients and stir well.
2. Add in the rest of the ingredients, except for milk and raspberries, and combine until a thick batter is formed.
3. Stir in the raspberries and add one tbsp. of milk. Add extra milk if the batter gets too thick. Place in microwave and cook for 1 to 2 minutes. Should come out gooey in the center. If you overcook, it will become dry.

Oven Directions

1. Heat oven up to 180C.
2. Oil an oven-proof ramekin. Add the prepared batter and put in the oven for 10-12 minutes, or until done.

9. Keto Avocado Brownies

Prep. Time: 10 minutes

Cook Time: 30 minutes

Servings: 12 squares

Nutrition as per serving:

155kcal / 14g fat / 13g carbs / 10g fiber / 4g protein = 2.8g net carbs

Ingredients

- Avocado, mashed 1 cup

- Vanilla 1/2 tsp

- Cocoa powder 4 tbsp.

- Refined coconut oil (or ghee, butter, lard, shortening) 3 tbsp.

- Eggs 2

- Lily's chocolate chips melted 1/2 cup (100 g)

Dry Ingredients

- Blanched almond flour 3/4 cup

- Baking soda 1/4 tsp

- Baking powder 1 tsp

- Salt 1/4 tsp

- Erythritol 1/4 cup (see sweetener note *1)

- Stevia powder 1 tsp (see sweetener note *1)

Directions

1. Heat the oven up to 350F/ 180C.

2. Sift together the dry ingredients in a small bowl and stir.

3. Place the Peeled avocados in a food processor and process until smooth.

4. One by one, add all the wet ingredients into the food processor, processing every few seconds

5. Now include the dry ingredients into the food processor and blend until combined.

6. Line a parchment paper in a baking dish (of 12"x8") and transfer the batter into it. Spread evenly and put in the heated oven. Cook for 30 minutes or the center springs back to touch. It should be soft to touch.

7. Remove from oven, set aside to cool fully before cutting into 12 slices.

10. Low Carb-1 minute Cinnamon Roll Mug Cake

Prep. Time: 1 minute

Cook Time: 1 minute

Servings: 1 serving

The serving size is 1mug

Nutrition as per serving:

132kcal / 4g fat / 6g carbs / 2g fiber / 25g protein = 4g net carbs

Ingredients

• Protein powder, vanilla flavor 1 scoop

• Baking powder 1/2 tsp

• Coconut flour 1 tbsp.

• Cinnamon 1/2 tsp

• Granulated sweetener 1 tbsp.

• Egg 1 large

- Almond milk, unsweetened 1/4 cup

- Vanilla extract 1/4 tsp

- Granulated sweetener 1 tsp

- Cinnamon 1/2 tsp

For the glaze

- Coconut butter melted 1 tbsp.

- Almond milk 1/2 tsp

- Cinnamon a pinch

Directions

1. Oil a microwave-proof mug. In a small bowl, add the protein powder, coconut flour, baking powder, sweetener, cinnamon and mix well.

2. Add in the egg and stir into the flour mixture. Include the vanilla extract and milk. If the batter is too dry, keep adding milk until a thick consistency is reached.

3. Pour this batter into the oiled mug. Sprinkle extra cinnamon and keto granulated sweetener over the top and swirl. Place in microwave and cook for 60 seconds, or till the center is just cooked. Do not overcook, or it will come out dry. Drizzle the glaze on top and enjoy!

4. Prepare glaze by mixing all ingredients and use.

11. Double Chocolate Muffins

Prep. Time: 10 minutes

Cook Time: 15 minutes

Servings: 12 muffins

The serving size is 1 muffin

Nutrition as per serving:

280 kcal / 27g fat / 7g carbs / 4g fiber / 7g protein = 3g net carbs

Ingredients

- Almond flour 2 cup
- Cocoa powder unsweetened 3/4 cup
- Swerve sweetener 1/4 cup
- Baking powder 1 1/2 tsp.
- Kosher salt 1 tsp.
- Butter melted 1 cup (2 sticks)
- Eggs 3 large
- Pure vanilla extract 1 tsp.
- Dark chocolate chips, sugar-free (like lily's) 1 cup

Directions

1. Heat oven up to 350° and line cupcake liners in a muffin tin. In a big bowl, stir together almond flour, Swerve, cocoa powder, salt and baking powder. Include eggs, melted butter and vanilla and mix until combined.

2. Stir in the chocolate chips.

3. Pour batter equally in muffin cups and bake for 12 minutes or until the muffin top springs back to touch.

Chapter 4- Keto Fat Bombs

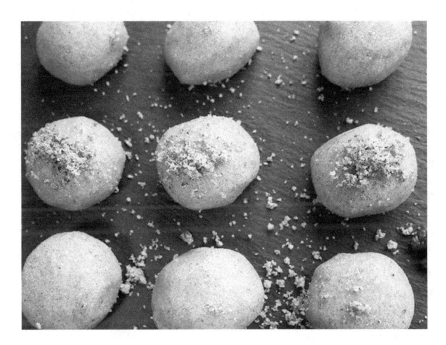

1. Cheesecake Fat Bombs

Prep. Time: 5 minutes

Servings: 24Fat Bombs

The serving size is 1 Fat Bomb

Nutrition as per serving:

108kcal / 12g fat / 1g carbs / 1g fiber / 1g protein = 0g net carbs

Ingredients

- Heavy Cream 4 oz.

- Cream cheese at room temperature 8 oz.

- Erythritol 2-3 tbsp.

- Coconut oil or butter 4 oz.

- Vanilla extracts 2tsp.

- Baking chocolate or coconut for decorating

Directions

1. In a big mixing bowl, add all the ingredients and mix for 1-2 minutes with an electric mixer until well combined and creamy.

2. Spoon mixture into an unlined or lined mini cupcake tin. Chill for 1-2 hours in the refrigerator or freezer for about 30 minutes.

3. Take out from the cupcake tins and store them in a sealed container. It can be refrigerated for up to two weeks.

2. Brownie Fat Bombs

Prep. Time: 15 minutes

Servings: 16 fat bombs

The serving size is 2 fat bombs

Nutrition as per serving:

174 kcal / 16g fat / 4g carbs / 2g fiber / 3g protein = 2g net carbs

Ingredients

- Ghee 1/4 cup

- Cocoa butter 1 oz.

- Vanilla extract 1/2 tsp

- Salt 1/4 tsp

- Raw cacao powder 6 tbsp.

- Swerve Sweetener powdered 1/3 cup

- Water 2 tbsp.

- Almond butter 1/3 cup

- Nuts, chopped (optional) 1/4 cup

Directions

1. melt the cocoa butter and ghee together In a heat-safe bowl placed over a pot of simmering water,

2. Add in the sweetener, cacao powder, salt and vanilla extract. This mixture will be smooth and thin.

3. Stir in the water and beat the mixture till it thickens to the consistency of a thick frosting.

4. Mix in the nut butter with a rubber spatula. The mixture will look like cookie dough. Mix in the coarsely chopped nuts.

5. Shape into 1 inch sized balls (will make about 16) and chill until firm.

3. Coffee Fat Bombs

Prep. Time: 10 minutes

Servings: 8 Fat Bombs

The serving size is 1 Fat Bomb

Nutrition as per serving:

140 kcal / 14g fat / 4g carbs / 2g fiber / 1.5g protein = 2g net carbs

Ingredients

- Cream Cheese, Full-fat 8 Oz.

- Butter Unsalted, ½ cup (1 Stick)

- Instant Coffee 1 to 2 Tbsps.

- Chocolate Chips, Low Carb, heaped ¼ Cup

- Confectioners Erythritol heaped ⅓ Cup

- Cocoa Powder, Unsweetened 1½ Tbsp.

Directions

1. In a large bowl, place the butter and cream cheese (both should be at room temperature)

2. Combine them with an electric mixer until smooth.

3. Then include all the remaining ingredients in the bowl, blending until well-combined

4. Scoop out the batter with a tablespoon or a cookie scoop to make around 12 bombs. Place them on a baking sheet lined with parchment. Chill for about 3 hours.

4. Peanut Butter Fat Bombs

Prep. Time: 10 minutes

Servings: 12 fat bombs

The serving size is 1/2 fat bomb

Nutrition as per serving:

247 kcal / 24.3g fat / 3.2g carbs / 1.2g fiber / 3.6g protein = 2g net carbs

Ingredients

For fat bomb

- Natural peanut butter (no sugar) 3/4 cup

- Coconut oil (melted) 1/2 cup

- Vanilla extract 1 tsp.

- Liquid stevia 3 – 4 drops

- Sea salt 1/4 tsp.

For Ganache

- Coconut oil 6 tbsp.
- Cocoa powder 1 tbsp.
- Liquid stevia 1 – 2 drops

Directions

1. Mix the peanut butter, coconut oil, vanilla extract, salt, and liquid stevia together in a small mixing bowl, beat until creamy and smooth.
2. Line muffin paper cups in a six-cup-muffin tray. Fill each cup with about 3 tbsp. of the peanut butter mixture.
3. Refrigerate for about 1 hour to solidify.
4. Meanwhile, beat together the ingredients for Ganache until it's silky.
5. Drizzle about one tbsp. of the chocolate ganache on every fat bomb.
6. Chill for about 30 minutes and enjoy.

5. Cream Cheese Pumpkin Spiced Fat Bombs

Prep. Time: 10 minutes

Servings: 12 Fat Bombs

The serving size is 1 Fat Bomb

Nutrition as per serving:

80 kcal / 7.5g fat / 2g carbs / 0.25g fiber / 1.5g protein = 1.75g net carbs

Ingredients

- Pure pumpkin ⅔ cup

- Pumpkin pie spice ½ tsp

- Cream cheese, full-fat 8 oz.

- Butter melted 3 tbsps.

- Confectioner's erythritol 3 tbsps.

Directions

1. Place all the ingredients in a large bowl and mix with an electric mixer until combined.

2. Make 12 equal-sized balls from the dough. Place paper liners in a mini-muffin tin and place the PB cookie dough in the muffin tin.

3. Chill for a minimum of 2 hours

Note:

If the pumpkin pie spice is not available, make some with the following ingredients

¼ tsp cinnamon, a pinch of (each) - nutmeg, cloves, ginger and allspice.

6. Brownie Truffles

Prep. Time: 5 minutes

Cook Time: 5 minutes

Servings: 20 Truffles

The serving size is 1 Truffle

Nutrition as per serving:

97kcal / 8g fat / 5g carbs / 3g fiber / 4g protein = 2g net carbs

Ingredients

- Sticky sweetener, keto-friendly 1/2 cup of choice

- Homemade Nutella 2 cups
- Coconut flour 3/4 cup (or almond flour 1 ½ cup)
- Chocolate chips, sugar-free 2 cups

Directions

1. Combine the coconut/almond flour, sticky sweetener and chocolate spread in a big mixing bowl. Add a bit more syrup or liquid; if the mixture is too thick, it should become a creamy dough.
2. Place parchment paper on a large plate. Shape into small balls with your hands, and set on the plate. Chill.
3. Melt the sugar-free chocolate chips. Take the truffles from the refrigerator. Immediately, coat each truffle with the melted chocolate, making sure all are evenly coated.
4. Set back on the lined
5. Plate and chill until firm.

7. Coconut Strawberry Fat Bombs

Prep. Time: 10 minutes

Servings: 20 fat bombs

The serving size is 1fat Bomb

Nutrition as per serving:

132kcals / 14.3g fat / 0.9g carbs / 0g fiber / 0.4g protein = 0.9g net carbs

Ingredients

For Coconut base:

- Coconut cream 1 1/2 cups

- Coconut oil (melted) 1/2 cup

- Stevia liquid 1/2 tsp.

- Lime juice 1 tbsp.

For Strawberry topping:

- Fresh chopped strawberries 2 oz.

- Coconut oil (melted) 1/2 cup

- Liquid stevia 5 – 8 drops

Directions

Prepare the coconut base:

1. In a high-speed blender, place all the coconut base ingredients and blend them completely until combined and smooth.

2. Distribute the mixture evenly into an ice cube tray, muffin tray, or a candy mold, leaving room for the topping.

3. Chill in the freezer to set for about 20 minutes.

For the Strawberry topping:

1. In a blender, put all the ingredients for the strawberry topping, then blend until smooth.

2. When the base is set, spoon the strawberry mixture equally over each one.

3. Refrigerate the fat bombs for about 2 hours and enjoy.

8. Raspberry & White Chocolate Fat Bombs
Prep. Time: 5 minutes

Servings: 10-12 fat bombs

The serving size is 1 fat Bomb

Nutrition as per serving:

153kcal / 16g fat / 1.5g carbs / 0.4g fiber / 0.2g protein = 1.2g net carbs

Ingredients

- Cacao butter 2 oz.
- Coconut oil 1/2 cup
- Raspberries freeze-dried 1/2 cup
- Erythritol sweetener, powdered (like swerve) 1/4 cup

Directions

1. Place paper liners in a 12-cup muffin pan.
2. In a small pot, heat the cacao butter and coconut oil on low flame until melted completely. Take off the pot from heat.
3. Blend the freeze-dried raspberries in a blender or food processor, or coffee grinder.
4. Include the sweetener and powdered berries into the pot, stirring to dissolve the sweetener.
5. Distribute the mixture evenly between the muffin cups. Don't worry if the raspberry powder sinks to the bottom. Just stir the mixture when pouring them into each mold to distribute the raspberry powder in each mold.
6. Chill until hard. Enjoy.

9. Almond Joy Fat Bombs (3 Ingredients)

Prep. Time: 2 minutes

Cook Time: 3 minutes

Servings: 24 cups

The serving size is 1 cup

Nutrition as per serving:

72kcal / 8g fat / 6g carbs / 4g fiber / 2g protein = 2g net carbs

Ingredients

• Coconut butter softened 1/4 cup

• Chocolate chips, sugar-free, divided 20 oz.

• Almonds 24 whole

Directions

1. Place muffin liners in a 24-cup mini muffin tin and put them aside.

2. Melt 3/4 of the sugar-free chocolate chips in a microwave-proof bowl. Distribute the chocolate mixture equally into all the muffin liners. Also, scrape down all the chocolate coated on the sides. Chill until firm.

3. When the chocolate is hard, spoon in the melted coconut butter evenly into every chocolate cup, leaving room for chocolate filling on top. Add in more softened coconut butter if needed.

4. Melt the rest of the chocolate chips and with it, cover each of the chocolate coconut cups. Place an almond on top of each cup and chill until firm.

10. Pecan pie fat bombs

Prep. Time: 15 minutes

Servings: 18 balls

The serving size is 2 balls

Nutrition as per serving

121 kcal / 12g fat / 3.8g carbs / 2.9g fiber / 2g protein = 0.9g net carbs

Ingredients

- Pecans, (or any nut) 1½ cup s
- Coconut butter, ¼ cup
- Coconut shredded ½ cup
- Chia seeds 2 tbsp.
- Pecan butter (or any nut butter) 2 tbsp.
- Flax meal 2 tbsp.
- Coconut oil 1tsp.
- Hemp seeds 2 tbsp.
- Vanilla extract ½tsp.
- Cinnamon 1½tsp.
- Kosher salt ¼tsp.

Directions

1. Add the ingredients altogether in a food processor. Process for a minute or two to break down the mixture. First, it will become powdery. Then it will stick together but remain crumbly.

2. Continue to process until the oils begin to expel a bit, and the mixture will begin to stick together easily –be cautious not to process excessively, or you will have nut butter.

3. Using a tablespoon or small cookie scooper, scoop to make equal pieces of the mixture. Roll them into balls with your hands placing them all on a large plate. Chill for about 30 mins.

4. Keep in a sealed container or a zip-lock bag in the freezer or refrigerator.

11. PB. Cookie Dough Fat Bomb

Prep. Time: 10 minutes

Servings: 12 Fat Bombs

The serving size is 1 Fat Bomb

Nutrition as per serving:

135kcal / 11g fat / 5g carbs / 3.5g fiber / 4g protein = 1.5g net carbs

Ingredients

• Lily's chocolate chips ⅓ cup

• Almond flour, superfine 1 cup

• Natural peanut butter 6 tbsps.

• Confectioner's erythritol 2 tbsps.

• Coconut oil (melted) 1 tbsps.

• Vanilla extract 1 tsp

• Salt, a pinch

Directions

1. Place all the ingredients in a large bowl and mix with a spoon until crumbly.

2. Form a dough ball with your hands.

3. Line parchment paper on a baking sheet. Scoop out equal-sized 12 cookie dough fat bombs.

4. Chill for about an hour

5. Once they are done setting, keep in a sealed bag in the fridge.

Conclusion

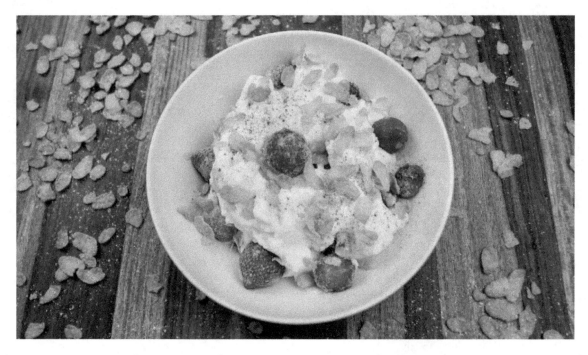

When going on a ketogenic diet, one retains modest protein consumption but increases their fat intake. The transition to a low-carb diet brings your body into a ketosis state, where fat is used for energy compared to carbohydrates.

It takes some time for fats to decompose through the digestive tract and delay the decomposition of the carbohydrates into sugar, maintain our blood sugar concentrations steady and allow us to feel satiated longer. Based on observational evidence, incorporating a tablespoonful of coconut oil into your diet every day may also result in lower weight.

You may also need to monitor the portion sizes, but as fat is intrinsically pleasing, having one for breakfast will help deter eating during meals.

When consuming high-fat meals, including keto fat bombs, you will further encourage weight reduction by decreasing appetite for the next meal. Be it fat bombs or cheesy waffles or any other hi fat low-carb dessert, they are a dieter's dream come true.

Following the keto diet can positively impact one's brain function.

Advantages of the ketogenic diet and fat bombs.

Keto fat bombs may be seen as a way to reduce sugar habits.

Ketogenic fat bombs are simple to produce, easy to keep, and easy to eat; they often need fewer ingredients than other foods.

Ketogenic fat bombs are tasty and have a broad variety of low-carb recipes.

Ketogenic fat bombs are quick to produce, are easy to store, and are ready to consume at any time.

In this book, you will find the best and easy to prepare keto cakes, chaffles, and yummy high-fat recipes that will fulfill your cravings for desserts after meals or snacks when you don't feel too hungry. Enjoy these recipes by yourself, or even better, share the joy with family and friends!

Intermittent Fasting for Women Over 60

The Science-Based Program for Seniors to Conquer and Keep a Young Body, Reset Your Metabolism and Activate Autophagy Above 60's

[11 Anti-Aging Exercises Included]

By

Stacey Bell

Table of Contents

INTRODUCTION

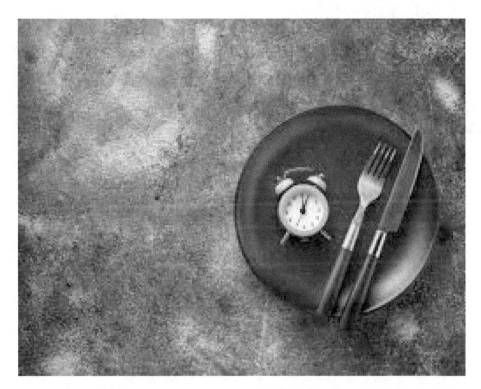

What exactly does intermittent fasting refer to? Almost all of us are familiar with the word fasting. The reasons people fast vary from one group to another. For some, it is a religious practice; they sacrifice food to commit to prayer. Others have no reason; they just lack food. In past societies, people would go out to the fields to work, and eat only when they rested.

Intermittent fasting is not among the fasting practices described above. It is neither a religious practice, nor is it driven by the lack of time or food - it is a choice. It is best described as an eating pattern that alternates between eating periods and fasting periods, with each period lasting a predetermined amount of time. For example, the 16:8 method has a fasting period of 16 hours and an eating period of 8 hours.

Note that it is not a diet but an eating pattern. Less is said about the foods you should eat, but more emphasis is put on when you eat them. Does this mean you can eat whatever you want? Unfortunately not. Just like anything else in life, you're going to get out what you put in. Clean eating is one of the three factors in the tripod to fat burning success. Does this mean you must live on chicken and broccoli? No of course not. We are humans and I believe in enjoying life, but as you already know moderation is the key here.

It is important to know that IF isn't some program that popped up from somewhere, will trend for a while, and disappear like most weight loss programs do. It has been around for a long time and has been popular for many years (even if you are learning about it just now). It is one of the leading health and fitness trends in the world today.

PART ONE

Knowledge (The Science-Based Program for Seniors to Conquer and Keep a Young Body)

How Fat is Stored & Burnt

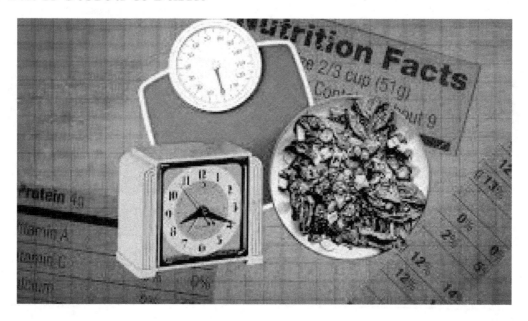

Intermittent fasting has been tried and found to be a powerful fat burning and weight loss tool. But how exactly does it work? Before delving into how IF works it's important to understand some key factors:

➢ How the body stores energy

➢ How the body uses energy

➢ Your hormones role in this process

The body is either in a state of storing energy or burning energy. There is no middle ground.

What does this mean? Well basically if you're not burning glucose (sugar) you're storing it as either glycogen or fat. Does this mean you need to be constantly working out? Short answer- no. In fact, exercise is only 10% - 15% of the weight loss equation (more about that later). Your body burns energy in a variety of different ways. Even when you're stationary doing absolutely nothing your body expends energy as it completes functions required for living. This is what RMR or BMR refers to. However, even though your cells might be using glucose and burning energy, any excess will be stored. This would count as a state of storage.

Wait! If we're either storing sugar or burning it, logic would dictate less food and more exercise equals weight loss. It seems straight forward, right? If you're reading this you have most likely tried this approach to no avail. You either saw results in the beginning only to have them come to a grinding halt or you put it all back on when you returned to your normal lifestyle.

So, how do I lose weight then?? To get a better picture we need to understand two principles:

1.   How glucose (sugar) is stored and burned, or used for energy.

2.   Our hormone's role in this process

How is energy stored?

The body can store energy in two ways; glycogen and fat.

Food (yum) is broken down into a variety of different macronutrients through digestion. These macronutrients are absorbed into the bloodstream and transported throughout the body to our cells to use for various functions. For example, Carbohydrates are broken down into Glucose (sugar), absorbed by the blood stream and sent to cells to use for energy. However, if there is excess glucose in the bloodstream (high blood sugar), it will be stored as glycogen through a process called Glycogenesis. The body can only store so much glycogen. Once these stores are full any excess glucose is stored as fat through a process called Lipogenesis.

How is energy used?

When our cells require more energy than the bloodstream can provide (low blood sugar) glycogen is turned back into glucose through a process called glycogenolysis. Our glycogen stores are slowly emptied to raise our blood sugar levels back to normal. When these stores are empty, fat will be broken down for energy in a process called lipolysis. Now we're burning fat Wahoo!

Summary

➢   Excess glucose will be turned into glycogen for storage, triggered by high blood sugar

➢   Once glycogen stores are full, excess glucose will be turned into fat for storage

➢   When blood sugar levels drop, glycogen will be turned back into glucose and added to the bloodstream

➢   When glycogen stores are emptied, fat will be broken down and released into the bloodstream for energy

Now you have a rough idea of how and why the body stores and uses energy, we will look at some key hormones that control this process.

Why Low-Calorie Diets Don't Work

Have you ever tried lowering your calories to lose weight? Did it work long term? Could you keep the weight you lost off? If you're reading this book, my guess is that it didn't, and you're not alone. Data from the UK show 1 in 124 obese women get results using this method, meaning the nutrition guidelines some professionals are following have a 99.5% fail rate. A quick goggle of what happened to the contestants on the hit TV series "The Biggest Loser" should be enough to put you off this method. This show is a classic example of why moving more and eating less only works in the short term, if at all. There is a reason there are few reunion shows. So why are low calorie diets flawed?

A study on 14 contestants on the biggest loser show revealed some alarming results six years after filming had finished. The initial results were impressive but as the study showed, they were short lived. Below are results of some of the factors tested.

Weight

- Average weight before filming: 328 lb./ 148 kg

- Average weight after 30 weeks on the show: 199 lb./ 90 kg

- Average weight six years after final: 290 lb./131 kg

As you can see, contestants lost a massive amount of weight during filming, but struggled to maintain the weight loss over a long period of time.

One of the 14 who participated in the study managed to keep the weight off. That's over a 95% fail rate! So why is this?

Check out the results below showing contestants Resting metabolic rate (RMR).

Resting Metabolic Rate

RMR reflects the amount of energy or calories the body burns to stay alive without movement.

In some places this is measured in BMR or basal metabolic rate.

RMR is responsible for around 70% of your entire metabolism which is why the results below are shocking.

- Average RMR before filming: 2,607 kcal burned / day.

- Average RMR after 30 weeks on the show: 1,996 kcal burned / day.

- Average RMR six years after final weigh-in: 1,903 kcal burned / day.

As you can see, even though contestants put around 70% of their initial weight back on, their RMR did not raise back to its levels pre- filming. It stayed around 700 calories lower a day! This means to lose the same amount of weight second time round; contestants would need to eat 700 less calories than they did on the show. Considering the original diet consists of 1200 - 1500 calories with 90 minutes of exercise six days a week. This would be near impossible.

So why did the contestants RMR stay so low even when they put the weight back on?

Metabolic adaptation

I mentioned BMR (basal metabolic rate) and RMR (resting metabolic rate) earlier. These both refer to how much energy (calories) your body uses to live without action and make up roughly 70% of your entire metabolism. When you sit in caloric deficit, the bodies BMR/RMR will slowly drop as it enters starvation mode, meaning it will burn less calories. Basically, your metabolism slows down. This is an important reaction through times of famine. The body doesn't want to use its stored energy, and naturally uses incoming energy sparingly. This is not beneficial when the aim is everlasting, sustainable weight loss. When you start dieting in this manner and increase your exercise you will generally only see results at the start before your body's metabolism adjusts for the lack of food. Once it adjusts, your results become stagnant and often times after frustration people give up and all the weight comes piling back on. If you're lucky your RMR/BMR will rise with the weight gain, ensuring you only end up putting back on what you lost, but constant yo-yo dieting could lead to a lower metabolism meaning you will struggle to lose weight and could even end up the heaviest you've ever been!

So, if eating too little causes this, you're probably wondering how not eating at all over a period of time could be any better right? Keep reading to see why.

Intermittent fasting vs Low calorie diets

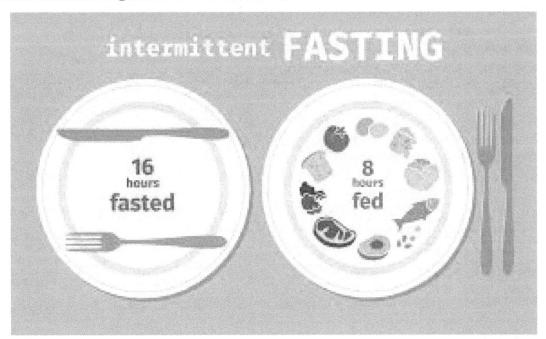

Low calorie diets simply don't cause the hormone adaptations fasting does. Remember those hormones we covered earlier in the book? They are the key to weight loss and your salvation. Remember how we need the help of hormones such as glucagon and HGH to stimulate the liver and fat cells to break down stored energy? As we now know they're triggered by low blood sugar levels. This is accomplished during the fasted period. Other hormones I haven't mentioned for simplicity's sake are also stimulated during this window to prevent metabolism drops associated with low calorie diets. Low calorie diets still include eating, and every time we eat our blood sugar levels are going to rise which triggers.........Insulin! As you now know, insulin is a storage hormone. So even though you might be consuming low calories, your lowered metabolism plus this little guy equals stored fat. Nothing turns off HGH like high blood sugar levels and insulin which ruins your chance to maintain muscle mass.

Summary

• Low calorie dieting could ruin your metabolism making maintainable weight loss near impossible

• Maintainable weight loss relies heavily on hormone adaptation

• Fasting stimulates key hormones for metabolism retention, muscle preservation, and fat burning

WHAT YOU SHOULD WEIGH

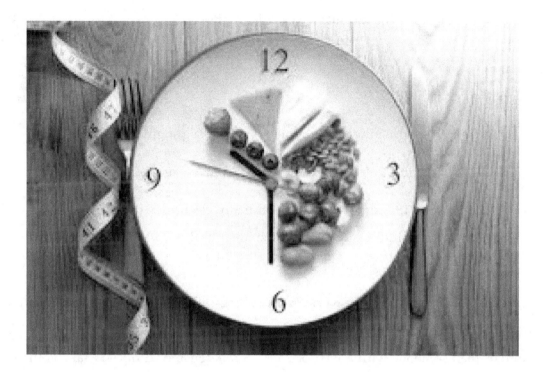

Before you embark on a fasting program for weight loss, let me help you establish what you should weigh. For many people, women in particular, the figure we think of as "ideal" is far removed from what is realistic, or even healthy. I could go on and blame the media or the fashion industry. We all know that argument and, yes, it's partly true.

Ironically, where I learned about fasting in India, the thought of using fasting to get slim would be abhorrent, as being skinny is associated with poverty and lower social castes. Fasting should never be used to strive for a body that's slimmer than is healthy – the size zero craze being a case in point. The less body fat you have to lose, the more you need to ensure that fasting is not over- done since weight loss is a guaranteed side-effect.

BODY MASS INDEX (BMI)

Healthy weight ranges are especially useful if you're already light for your frame

– you've probably heard of BMI, which gives an indication of how healthy your current weight is in proportion to your height. The formula for calculating BMI is:

BMI = weight (kg) ÷ height (m)2

(in other words, your weight in kilograms divided by your height in meters squared).

If math isn't your strong point, you can find out your BMI using an online calculator.

A healthy BMI is between 18.5 and 24.9. Although many celebrities have a BMI below 18.5, this simply isn't healthy. Some studies suggest that the ideal BMI is 23 for men and 21 for women – particularly if it's a long and healthy life you're after.

However, if your BMI is, say, 25 you won't become magically healthier by losing 450g (1lb) and dieting down to a BMI of 24.9. In fact, it's perfectly possible for someone with a BMI of 27 to be much healthier than someone with a BMI of 23. That's because BMI doesn't take your body fat, waist circumference, eating habits or lifestyle into account. An example of this could be a professional rugby player who's heavier than average simply because he or she is very muscular. There's nothing unhealthy about having lots of muscle, but the BMI scale might say he or she is overweight or even obese. In contrast, a chain-smoker who lives on diet drinks and never exercises can have a so-called "healthy" BMI. Who do you think is healthier?

A BMI of 30 or above is considered "obese". A 2008 study by researchers at the Mayo Clinic in the USA, involving over 13,000 people, found that 20.8 percent of men and 30.7 percent of women were obese according to the BMI scale. But when they used the World Health Organization gold standard definition of obesity – measuring body fat percentage – 50 percent of the men and 62.1 percent of the women were classified as obese. (In other words, you can have a healthy BMI and an unhealthy level of body fat.) What this means is that the athlete who's unfairly classed as "obese" is the exception rather than the rule. Unless you're an avid weight-lifter or sportsperson, or you have an extremely physical job, the BMI scale isn't likely to tell you that you need to lose weight if you don't. If your BMI is well over 25, don't worry. Medical experts agree that losing 5–10 percent of your starting weight is a sensible and realistic initial goal that will have lasting health benefits.

Therefore, when it comes to the BMI scale, it is worth calculating your BMI before deciding on a weight loss goal, especially if you only have a little weight to lose, but it definitely shouldn't be the only thing you think about.

BODY FAT PERCENTAGE

What's great about monitoring your body fat percentage is that it gives you a better understanding of what's going on inside your body as you lose weight. Sustainable weight loss is best achieved through a combination of good nutrition and an active lifestyle. The thing is, when you start exercising more, you often gain muscle mass.

It can be demotivating to step onto the scales and see that your overall weight hasn't changed in spite of all your hard work. But because muscle is denser than fat, you can look slimmer and achieve health benefits without actually losing weight. To track changes in your body fat, you need to invest in body composition scales which enable you to track your progress by measuring changes in your muscle mass, body fat and hydration. Gyms often have high- quality versions of these scales if you don't want to buy your own.

Body composition scales are also helpful because if you notice that your muscle mass is decreasing as rapidly as your body fat, this suggests that you've cut your energy intake too dramatically. For most people, it's realistic to lose 450–900g (1–2lb) of body fat per week. If you're losing much more than this, the chances are you're eating into your muscle mass. Body composition scales can alert you to this before you've risked damaging your health.

In women, it's normal for hydration levels to fluctuate along with the menstrual cycle. Again, measuring weight alone doesn't enable you to track these changes. By using the body composition scales at a similar time of day, and recording changes throughout the month, you can get a clearer understanding of the times you're gaining body fat, and when it's simply a matter of fluid retention.

Sophisticated body composition monitors also enable you to track abdominal fat. Remember, not all fat is created equal, and abdominal fat is concentrated around your vital organs, posing the biggest health risk. You can be a "healthy" weight, and have high levels of abdominal fat – being aware of this can give you the motivation you need to address your eating habits and activity level.

The scales use a weak electric current to differentiate between fat, muscle, fluid and bone – we won't go into too much detail here as different brands have different features. As a guide, if you're an ordinary adult, and not an athlete or aspiring fitness model, you should be aiming for the following body fat percentages:

AGE	MALE	FEMALE
20–39	8–20%	21–33%
40–59	11–22%	23–34%
60+	13–25%	24–36%

WHY TRADITIONAL DIETING MAKES YOU HUNGRY

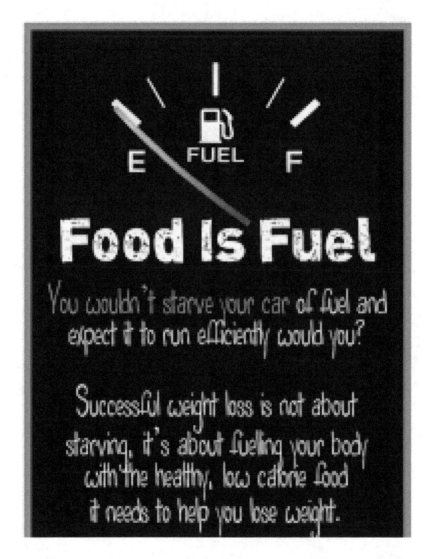

Going on a traditional diet without adequate energy intake for long periods of time can make your metabolic rate plummet and your appetite soar. Say you reduce your calories to below 1,000 a day for a number of weeks to fit into a party dress, the chances are you'll feel hungry and fed up much of the time, and as soon as the party starts, you'll dive head first into all the foods you've been avoiding, re-gaining that lost weight in no time! This, in a nutshell, sums up the seesaw of the diet industry.

The real trick is to keep your body feeling fuller for longer. I'm not talking about choosing one ready-meal over another, it's about understanding how to manage hunger so you naturally eat less most of the time. Please note, I don't say all of the time. Special events and over-indulging every now and then are good for the soul.

In tandem with a good diet overall, fasting can be used to retrain your hunger without the need for appetite suppressants or dodgy supplements. When you begin to fast, you will feel hungry at your usual meal times. However, if you choose not to eat at that time, the peaks and troughs of hunger start to level out. All this happens without a decrease in metabolic rate. It doesn't take a genius to recognize that if you feel hungry less often, you'll eat less and therefore lose weight. There's a biological explanation for this. Feelings of hunger and satiety (feeling full) are controlled by two main hormones produced within the body, ghrelin (even the word sounds hungry) and leptin. This dynamic duo of hormones has a powerful effect on how much food you eat and how much of what you've consumed you "burn off".

GHRELIN

This hormone seems pretty straightforward. When your stomach's empty, it sends out some ghrelin to tell an area of your brain, the hypothalamus, that you ought to be eating. You then feel ravenous. But research published in the American Journal of Physiology suggests that ghrelin levels also rise in anticipation of eating – you get hungry partly because you're expecting a meal, not just because you have an empty stomach.

On a traditional diet, you get a peak of ghrelin before every meal – but because you don't eat as much as you'd really like to, you never feel fully satisfied. When you're fasting, your ghrelin levels still rise, but anecdotal evidence suggests that over time your body finds this sensation easier to get used to, probably because of the changes in your meal patterns. There's also a theory that a nutritionally poor diet (think additive-packed "diet" meals) sends ghrelin rocketing faster than a nutrient-dense plan like the ones I recommend.

LEPTIN

This hormone is a little more complicated. You'll sometimes hear leptin referred to as a "master regulator" of fat metabolism. There are even whole diet books devoted to it.

Leptin is made by the fat cells – put simply, the more fat you have, the more leptin is produced. Like ghrelin, it sends a signal to the hypothalamus, but with the opposite effect. Leptin is supposed to maintain your body fat at a healthy level by telling you to stop eating when you start to gain too much fat. We all know it doesn't really work like that in practice – if it did, no one would be overweight. So, what happens?

Well, leptin also increases when you overeat – especially stodgy, carbohydrate-rich meals. This is because its release is triggered by insulin, which responds to an increase in blood glucose after a meal. So, if you're constantly eating without a proper break, your leptin levels will always be high. At first this is good – it should signal to your brain that it's time to put down that muffin – but it can lead to a very dangerous vicious circle. The theory is that, over time, too much leptin leads to the brain becoming resistant to its effects. As your brain stops recognizing what leptin is trying to tell it, you end up feeling hungry all the time, and are never satisfied by even the biggest meal.

WHY MOST DIETS FAIL

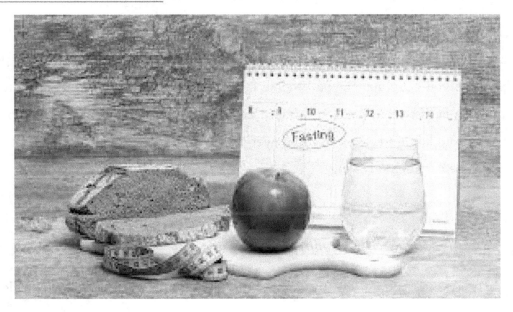

This probably isn't the first book about weight loss you've ever read. I often say I've been down the diet road myself so many times that I could be a tour guide. If you're asking yourself why fasting is going to be any different, here are the facts you need to know:

• "Yo-yo" dieting is the bane of many people's lives, but even if you've lost and gained weight countless times, recent research has shown that it's possible to lose weight safely without messing up your metabolism.

• Burning off more calories than you eat is the only way to lose weight – and the simple truth is that you will lose weight if you manage to keep the number of calories you eat below the amount you burn off… boring but true.

There are hundreds of different ways to create a calorie deficit – as evidenced by the huge diet book, diet shake, diet bar and "miracle" weight-loss supplement industry. But there are two main reasons why diets never tend to live up to their expectations, especially as you get closer to your goal weight:

1   _Traditional diet misrepresent the calories in/calories out equation_.

We've all heard that 450g (1lb) of fat is roughly equal to 3,500 calories, so the traditional calorie-counting approach is to cut calories by 500–1,000 per day in order to lose 450–900g (1–2lb) per week. The trouble is, as you get slimmer you become lighter and that actually reduces the number of calories you burn at rest (your basal metabolic rate). So, in traditional weight-loss plans, weight loss is initially rapid but tends to slow down over time, even if you maintain that original calorie deficit. This can be very demotivating.

2   _It's sticking to your chosen approach that's often the hard part._

Even if you get your calories exactly right, how boring does counting every calorie get? Demotivation – either as a result of not seeing the numbers on the scales going down as quickly as they were, or boredom – can lead to lapses, which slow down the rate of weight loss even further. When you go back to your old eating habits – surprise, surprise – you'll gain all the weight back, and a little more, as a result of the natural dip in basal metabolic rate (calorie burn) caused by your initial weight loss.

PART TWO

Action (Reset Your Metabolism)

HOW FASTING MAKES A DIFFERENCE

FASTING MAY BOOST METABOLIC RATE

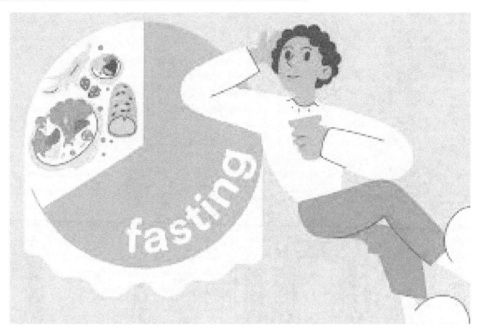

You're probably thinking, "If I start starving myself, won't that be worse for my metabolism?" First of all, fasting is not starving yourself, and don't worry that eating less often will damage your metabolism. Losing weight naturally slows your basal metabolic rate (the number of calories you burn at rest) in proportion to the amount of weight you lose, no matter which method you use. This is because your daily energy (calorie) needs are directly related to your age, height, gender and weight, in particular your lean body mass (muscle). It doesn't mean that eating more often will fire up your metabolism.

You'll hear over and over again that after a night of sleep, your metabolism has ground to a halt and you need to eat breakfast to stoke your metabolic fire. The idea that "breakfast boosts metabolism" is simply not true – it hasn't been backed up by research at all. The breakfast myth is based on the "thermic effect of food". Around 10 percent of our calorie burn comes from the energy that we use to digest, absorb and assimilate the nutrients in our meals. Roughly speaking, if you eat a 350-calorie breakfast, you'll burn 35 calories in the process. But notice that you've eaten 315 extra calories to burn that 35. No matter what time of day you eat, you'll burn off around 10 percent of the calories in your food through the thermic effect of food. So, whether you eat your breakfast at 7am, 10am or never, if you eat roughly the same amount and types of food overall, its effect on your metabolism will be the same.

In fact, all the research on fasting seems to show that eating less often could actually boost your metabolic rate. In one British study conducted at the University of Nottingham, a two-day fast boosted participants' resting metabolic rate by 3.6 percent. In another study by the same research group, 29 healthy men and women fasted for three days. After 12–36 hours, there was a significant increase in basal metabolic rate, which returned to normal after 72 hours. The exact mechanisms for why this happens aren't clear.

FASTING INCREASES FAT BURN

What is clear is that more of the calories you use for fuel during fasting come from your fat stores. Scientists can estimate what proportion of your energy is coming from fats and carbohydrates by measuring the amount of oxygen inhaled and the amount of carbon dioxide exhaled in your breath. The higher the proportion of oxygen to carbon dioxide, the more fat you're burning. As part of the same Nottingham study, findings proved that the proportion of energy obtained from fat rose progressively over 12–72 hours, until almost all the energy being used was coming from stored fat. This is incredible news really!

We're so often told to "breakfast like a king, lunch like a prince and dine like a pauper" with a view to becoming healthy, wealthy and wise. This is usually explained by telling us that breakfast kick-starts the metabolism – but it turns out that eating breakfast doesn't boost your fat-burning potential at all. In a small study on breakfast-eaters – published in the British Journal of Nutrition – a 700-calorie breakfast inhibited the use of fat for fuel throughout the day. Put simply, when we eat carbohydrates, we use it for fuel, and this prevents our bodies tapping into our stubborn stored fat. Constant grazing might be what's keeping fat locked away in your belly, bum or thighs – and fasting is one way to release it.

FASTING MAINTAINS LEAN MUSCLE

The more muscle you have, the more calories you burn at rest. And before you say you don't want big muscles, another way to put that is: the less muscle you lose as you drop in weight, the less your basal metabolic rate falls as you move toward your goal weight. (Remember, your basal metabolic rate is the rate at which you burn calories, so it's really important in order to make staying in shape easier in the long term.) Besides, muscle takes up less room than fat. So, a person with good lean muscle mass will take a smaller dress size or use a narrower belt notch than someone who doesn't have it.

Fasting is better than plain old calorie restriction when it comes to maintaining lean body mass. This is largely because fasting triggers the release of growth hormone (GH), which encourages your body to look for other fuel sources instead of attacking its muscle stores. This is thought to be a survival advantage – back when humans were hunter gatherers it wouldn't have made sense for our muscle mass to reduce when food was scarce – we needed strong legs and arms to hunt down our dinner!

In one study carried out by researchers at Intermountain Medical Center in the USA, participants were asked to fast for 24 hours. During this time, GH levels rose by a whopping 1,300 percent in women and 2,000 percent in men.

Many other studies have investigated the effects of fasting on GH. Like other hormones, GH levels rise and fall throughout the day and night. They tend to be highest at the beginning of a good night's sleep, when our stomachs are empty but our bodies are hard at work repairing in preparation for a new day. Larger or more frequent bursts of GH are released when we continue to fast and also when we take part in vigorous exercise.

GH acts by sending a signal to our fat cells to release some of their contents into the bloodstream. This enables us to use more fat for fuel, instead of burning mainly carbohydrates for energy. GH is also thought to maintain concentrations of another hormone, insulin-like growth factor (IGF-1), which helps our muscles to build more protein.

This is totally different to what happens when you simply cut calories without changing how often you eat. When you hear people saying you should eat little and often to maintain your blood glucose levels, what they're telling you to do, in actual fact, is to avoid this state. This is because whenever you top up your blood glucose levels through eating, your body releases insulin to compensate, and GH levels never get a boost when insulin is around.

It's important to note that more isn't necessarily better when it comes to GH – what's key is resetting the balance between GH release (which happens in the fasted state) and insulin release (which happens in the fed state, however small your meal) in order to stimulate fat loss without losing lean muscle. You never need to fear growing giant muscles as a result of fasting – GH is released in waves and goes back to normal levels quickly as soon as your body has released enough fat to burn.

As mentioned earlier, if you're already slim, it's especially important not to overdo it when fasting. Research published in the academic journal Obesity Research shows that within just two days of complete fasting, there's a dramatic increase in the use of muscle for fuel in people who are already a healthy weight. This is because they have less fat available to burn overall. Perhaps the advice for people who are already svelte but who want to fast for health benefits is to fast little and often rather than to eat little and often.

FASTING PATTERNS GIVE YOU ENERGY WHEN YOU NEED IT

Alongside maintaining your muscle mass to reduce the dip in your metabolic rate that happens as you lose weight, fasting may help with stubborn weight in other ways.

There's a theory that the reduction in calorie burn typically seen after following a calorie-restricted diet may be related more to changes in activity level than to basal metabolic rate. When you're only eating, say, 1,200 calories day after day, it may be difficult to maintain the energy levels and motivation to exercise. But following an intermittent fasting pattern means that you can concentrate your workouts around the times when you're eating. More energy means a tougher workout – and more calorie burn overall.

COMMON QUESTIONS AND ANSWERS

Q   Isn't "not eating" dangerous?

A   It's very important to establish that fasting is not starvation, which, of course, is dangerous. What I'm talking about is the health benefits of increasing the gaps between meals or eating less from time to time.

Some people who are fully signed up to the merry-go-round of traditional dieting will argue that not eating is likely to induce a low-blood-sugar or "hypo" episode. Feeling faint, clammy and unable to concentrate are typical symptoms, happily offset by a visit to the vending machine or, for the health- aware, a snack such as an oatcake or nuts and seeds. I'm not suggesting that snacking should be outlawed – most of the time, I'm more than happy to tuck right in. But fasting challenges the assertion that we can't survive, or even thrive, without five mini-meals a day.

I accept that challenging the blood-sugar story isn't going to win me any popularity prizes. However, the reality of what science is telling us today is that there's no medical consensus on the concept of low blood sugar. The vast majority of us are perfectly capable of regulating our blood glucose level and, although we may feel ravenous between meals, going without food for a few hours won't cause the blood glucose to plummet and, even if it does, our self-preserving mechanisms will kick into action long before we pass out. What this means is that insulin's countermeasure, glucagon, will kick in, releasing those locked-up glucose stores into the blood and bringing the glucose level back within its normal range.

A few words of warning, though... Diabetic "hypos" are a different thing altogether, of course, and can be very dangerous, but they are drug- induced. For people diagnosed as diabetic but who are not yet on insulin medication, fasting has proved promising. In a year-long study on intermittent fasting, the group who fasted every other day stayed off diabetes medication for significantly longer.

Q   Won't I feel light-headed and really hungry on a fast?

A   You might be worried that your blood sugar levels will dip too low between meals and that you'll feel faint and weak. But when you're not eating, other hormonal signals trigger your body to release glucose or make more. In one Swedish study by researchers at the Karolinska Institute, students who'd reported that they were sensitive to hypoglycemia (low blood sugar) felt irritable and shaky during a 24-hour fast, but there was actually no difference in their blood sugar levels – it may all have been in their minds.

It's true that your brain requires about 500 calories a day to keep the grey matter ticking over effectively. The brain's preferred fuel is glucose, which your liver stores around 400 calories-worth of at a time. In a longer fast, the body is forced to increase its production of ketone bodies, which act as a glucose-substitute for your brain. But in the short term, so long as you eat well before and after your fasting period, your body is perfectly able to produce enough glucose to keep your brain happy.

Q   Hang on a minute… My trainer told me that six small meals will fire up my metabolism and stop me feeling peckish. Who's right?

A This is one of those fitness and nutrition "truths" that has been repeated so many times, people are convinced that it's a fact. In one small study at the US National Institute on Aging, researchers found that people who ate only one meal a day did tend to feel hungrier than those who ate three. But beyond eating three meals a day, meal frequency doesn't seem to make a difference to hunger or appetite, so it comes down to what's actually easiest for you. A study published by the International Journal of Obesity showed that people who are overweight tend to snack more often.

Q   Can fasting change my shape?

A   For many women, that last bit of surplus weight is carried around the hips and thighs and it simply won't shift. To solve this problem, I suggest looking to the true body professionals.

According to noted intermittent-fasting expert Martin Berkhan, there's a good reason for this. All the cells in our body have "holes" in them known as receptors. To switch activity on and off in those cells, hormones or enzymes enter the receptors. Fat cells contain two types of receptor – beta 2 receptors, which are good at triggering fat burning, and alpha 2 receptors, which aren't. Guess which is mostly found in the fat stores of your lower body? Yes, our hips and thighs have nine times more alpha 2 receptors than beta.

Q   What about belly fat?

A   All over the Internet you'll see promises that you can get rid of belly fat in a matter of days by taking supplements. We all know that this is simply not true. Stubborn fat around the middle is linked to a number of factors – including stress, alcohol, lack of exercise and a diet high in refined carbohydrates.

Every time you eat something sweet or a refined carbohydrate such as biscuits or white bread, your blood sugar levels rise quickly, causing your pancreas to release the fat-storing hormone, insulin. If you spend the day going from sugary snack to sugary snack, and especially if you wash everything down with a couple of glasses of wine, your body ends up storing more of the calories you eat and you end up with that dreaded "muffin top"!

Stress + refined carbohydrates + alcohol = a recipe for belly fat, especially if you're unlucky enough to be genetically predisposed to weight gain around the middle.

Q   How does fasting help torch belly fat?

A   To burn belly fat, free fatty acids must first be released from your fat cells (this is called lipolysis) and moved into your bloodstream, then transferred into the mitochondria of muscle or organ cells, to be burned (a process known as beta-oxidation).

Glucagon (another pancreatic hormone that has pretty much an equal and opposite effect to insulin) rises around four to five hours after eating, once all the digested nutrients from your last meal have been stored or used up. The purpose of glucagon is to maintain a steady supply of glucose to the brain and red blood cells, which it achieves by breaking down stored carbohydrates and leftover protein fragments in the liver. It also activates hormone-sensitive lipase, which triggers the release of fat from the fat cells, allowing other cells to be fueled by fat as opposed to glucose.

When you're fasting, belly fat can be turned into energy to keep your organs working effectively and, for example, to provide power to the muscles that hold you upright, as well as fueling muscle movement.

In contrast, when you're constantly grazing, your body doesn't need to release glucagon. Instead, the pancreas pumps out insulin, which also acts to maintain blood glucose levels within a narrow range. Insulin encourages the fat cells to keep their fat tightly locked up. Not only that, but any spare glucose that isn't required for energy and cannot be stored can actually be converted into fat.

Q   What else can I do to help get rid of belly fat?

A   Endurance exercise selectively reduces abdominal fat and aids maintenance of lean body mass, so it's great to do in combination with intermittent fasting. Choose a fasting method that will enable you to take regular exercise – gentle activity such as walking will help, but high-intensity training is even better.

Also, a very small recent study, carried out at the University of Oklahoma in the USA, found that quality protein intake was inversely associated with belly fat, so make sure you fuel up on lean proteins (which your fasting plans are rich in), when you are eating.

Q   What about losing that last 4.5kg (10lb)?

A   This is often the hardest weight to shift. Not only that, it tends to creep back over a matter of weeks after you've finally reached your target weight. A familiar story is the strict diet we follow to get into beach-body shape in time for a holiday: in all the years I've helped people to lose weight, I've lost count of the number of times I've heard people telling me that all their hard work was undone by two weeks of sun, sea and sangria!

Remember that losing weight is all about creating a calorie deficit. Here, fasting is acting in two different ways. First, fasting helps maintain calorie burn – so in theory you can eat more overall and still lose weight. Second, fasting might just be easier to stick to than a boring calorie-counting diet. And when it comes to beach bodies, remember that old saying "a change is as good as a rest". If you're bored of the approach you've taken to weight loss up to now, a short blast of fasting can help you achieve your goal weight without damaging your metabolism.

FASTING AND CANCER

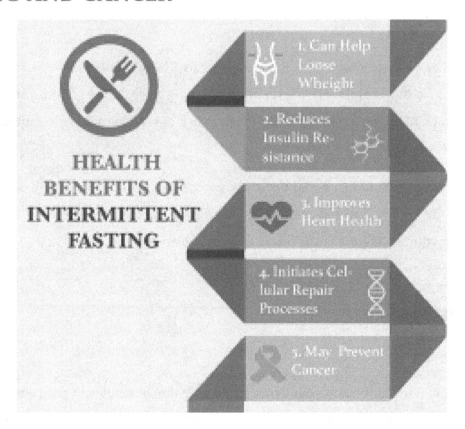

Fasting is considered to be an alternative or complementary treatment for cancer in certain sectors of complementary medicine, and has been popularized by a naturopathic doctor called Max Gerson. However, my focus is not on fasting as a stand-alone treatment but rather on exciting evidence about fasting in cancer prevention and the encouraging results from trials involving fasting during cancer treatment, particularly chemotherapy.

There's evidence that intermittent fasting, and calorie restriction more generally, fights the growth and spread of cancer cells in animals. Often when we read about research on animals, it seems so compelling that we want to see if the same thing will work for us. However, research is so much less likely to be done on humans as, rightly or wrongly, ethics committees are often reluctant to approve the same types of study that are done on animals. As discussed above, in experiments on laboratory animals, diets with 25 percent fewer calories have shown a positive link with longer, healthier life spans. So far there's little empirical study evidence to show the same effect in humans, yet anecdotal evidence is growing that restricting calories, and fasting, activates cell-protecting mechanisms. Research is also underway to find out whether alternate-day fasting can help reduce the risk of breast cancer.

In studies on mice with cancer, fasting appears to improve survival rates after chemotherapy. Hearing of the effects of these animal studies by Valter Longo, ten cancer patients took it upon themselves to try fasting before chemotherapy. The results were published in the medical journal *Aging*. Of these ten, the majority experienced fewer side-effects as a result of fasting than those eating normally, and the authors concluded that fasting for two to five days before chemotherapy treatment appeared to be safe. This work has yet to be taken to a truly meaningful empirical testing on humans, but it's understandable that cancer patients are excited by the potential of calorie restriction and fasting, not least by it helping the body to mitigate the effects of cancer treatment and specifically chemotherapy.

DETOXING

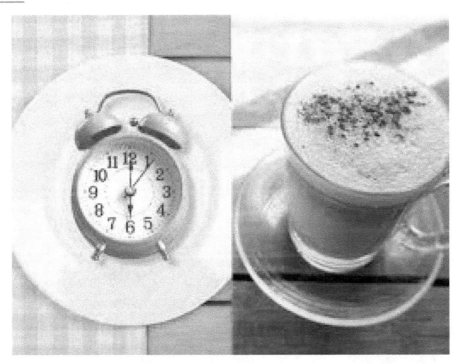

Personally, I no longer like the word "detox". It's been used and abused by marketeers in their quest to sell, sell, sell fancy products, when, in fact, detoxing is something that the body does naturally every hour of the day. However, until someone comes up with a better word, "detox" will have to do.

HOW WE BECOME TOXIC

A toxin is anything that has a detrimental effect on cell function or structure. Toxins are materials that our bodies cannot process efficiently. Over time they build up and, as a result, our systems function below par, leaving us drained, tired and frequently ill. People become "toxic" in many ways – through diet, lifestyle and the environment, as a natural by-product of metabolism, and through genetic lineage. Stress and harmful emotions can also create a kind of toxic environment.

Toxins include, but are not limited to:

- Food additives, flavorings and colorings.

- Household and personal cleaning chemicals, which are both inhaled and absorbed via the skin.

- Agricultural chemicals, such as pesticides, fungicides and herbicides.

- Heavy metals, which occur naturally but are poisonous.

- Oestrogens, which enter the environment due to human usage of the contraceptive pill and HRT.

- Xeno-oestrogens, which are chemicals that mimic oestrogen.

…And here are the most common ways people become toxic on the inside:

- Eating a poor diet. This includes low-fiber foods, fried foods and foods tainted with synthetic chemicals. Unlike live foods (fresh fruits and vegetables), these lack the enzymes that assist proper digestion and assimilation, and the fiber or bulk that assists proper elimination. They're also void of essential vitamins, minerals and other basic nutrients.

• Eating too much. Over-eating puts a great amount of stress on our digestive system. The body must produce hydrochloric acid, pancreatic enzymes, bile and other digestive factors to process a meal. When we over-eat, the digestive system finds it hard to meet the demands placed upon it. The stomach bloats as the digestive system goes into turmoil. Foods aren't broken down properly and tend to lodge in the lower intestine. Vital nutrients are then not absorbed.

• Inadequate water intake. When the body isn't receiving enough water, toxins tend to stagnate, hindering all digestive and eliminative processes.

• Exposure to synthetic chemicals in food and environmental pollutants. A clean, strong system can metabolize and excrete many pollutants, but when the body is weak or constipated, they're stored as unusable substances. As more and different chemicals enter the body, they tend to interact with those already there, forming second-generation chemicals that can be far more harmful than the originals.

• Being stressed. Stress hinders proper digestion, absorption and elimination of foods.

• Overuse of antibiotics. Antibiotics have a damaging effect on the intestines, especially if they're taken for extensive periods of time. Reducing the use of unnecessary antibiotics will also help minimize the very real danger of bacterial resistance.

• Lack of exercise. This lowers metabolic efficiency, and without circulatory stimulation, the body's natural cleansing systems are weakened.

• Eating late at night. The human body uses sleep to repair, rebuild and restore itself. In essence, the body uses the sleeping hours to cleanse and build. When a person goes to sleep with a full stomach, the body isn't at rest but is busy digesting and processing food. In addition, the body requires gravity to assist the passage of food from the stomach down the digestive tract.

Q   If the body detoxes itself anyway, why bother to do anything further?

A   Just as your home or office can become dusty and dirty, so your body can become clogged up with toxins and waste matter from the environment. A healthy body is able to disarm toxins by breaking them down, storing them in fat tissue or excreting them. However, here's the crux – many, if not most, people are depleted in the nutrients needed to detox optimally, and chronic health problems, sluggishness and weight gain are common results.

If you've never given your digestion much thought, don't beat yourself up about being neglectful. Unlike the head or the tips of the fingers, the gut contains very few nerve endings. What this means is, we're not so aware when things aren't working well. When you have a headache, you feel every throbbing pulse and do something about it. In contrast, gut problems go unresolved and uncared for over long periods.

The good news is, when you improve digestion, a whole range of seemingly unrelated health issues can improve. For example, it's not only the job of the white blood cells (the leukocytes) to defend your body since the digestive system forms the basis of your immune system with the action of beneficial bacteria. Improving the ecology of the gut can be achieved with a juice fast and healthy diet.

USING A JUICE FAST TO DETOX

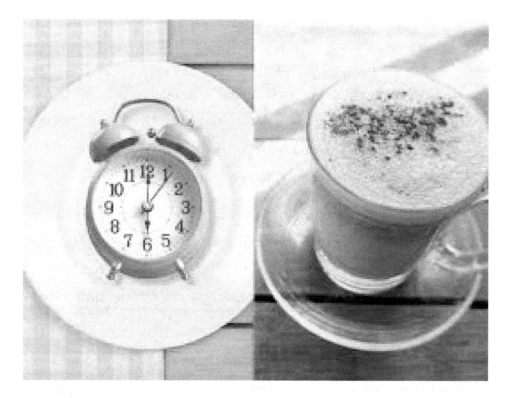

A juice fast stands head and shoulders above other fasting techniques in its self-healing effect and is often mentioned in the context of detoxing the body.

Juice fasting is based on consuming juices and broths only, whereas intermittent fasting adds lean protein and fat for the feeling of fullness. Studies have shown that eating as little as 10g (¼oz) of essential amino acids (found in high-quality proteins) can switch off autophagy. Therefore, a juice fast is best placed to give your body a good "spring clean" because juices are typically very low in protein.

The simple act of juicing a fruit or vegetable will help you absorb more of the nutrients from it. The caveat here is that you should make the juice fresh rather than drink pasteurized fruit juice from a carton or bottle. The process of juicing eliminates a lot of the fiber that needs to be digested. Cutting out the bulk and drinking only the juice means that you can very effectively hit your antioxidant targets in one small cup. Juice provides tiny "particles" of nutrients that are readily absorbed into the bloodstream.

Fresh juices provide a highly effective fast-track and – importantly – easy delivery mechanism for the body to absorb and process key vitamins, minerals and plant chemicals (phytonutrients) that are so beneficial to our health. A fresh juice contains a concentration of nutrients that have been separated from pulp, making it easier to consume what's required to assist the healing process. In essence, a fresh juice should be considered more of a body tonic than a tasty drink.

Q   Will I get withdrawal symptoms on a juice fast?

A   The folklore of fasting is littered with stories about the dramatic side-effects of a juice fast. This is usually because the contrast between the diet and lifestyle before and after is simply too great. Or, in some cases, the enterprising individual has decided to "retox", that is go on an almighty bender before entering detox – not a good idea.

One of the most dramatic side-effects I ever witnessed was when a client was coming off a 20-year-long diet cola habit during a juice-fasting retreat. Her symptoms were akin to what you'd expect from coming off a class-A drug. The rest of the detox group watched mesmerized at her descent from bubbly, bouncy guest on arrival to a sweating, vomiting, pale-faced shadow of her former self after just 24 hours of juicing. Even I was a little worried. Luckily, her troubled time was followed by a rapid and dramatic improvement two days later, at which point she declared that she felt "reborn" and would never touch a drop of cola again.

So, learn from my diet cola story and start with a transition diet. Fasting can be a challenge physically and psychologically. I recommend having at least three days on the Countdown Plan to prepare. Juice fasting should be undertaken for between one and five days for optimum results – usually once or twice a year. Any longer requires more management and should only be considered when there are adequate reserves (body fat) or if there's a specific medical condition. Some people find that weekend-long juice fasts four times a year are helpful.

Q   What are the most common side-effects of a juice fast?

A   Let me be frank – a juice fast isn't a good idea for a romantic break or naughty weekend away. During a juice fast the capacity of the eliminative organs – lungs, liver, kidneys, and skin – is greatly increased, and masses of accumulated metabolic wastes and toxins are quickly expelled. It's like pressing the accelerator button on your body's waste disposal unit. As part of the eliminative process, your body will be cleansing itself of old, accumulated wastes and toxins. This typically throws up symptoms such as offensive breath, dark urine, increased faecal waste, skin eruptions, perspiration and increased mucus. As I said, it's not exactly romantic!

Your digestive system is the star of a fasting program. Poor digestion can be a hidden cause of weight gain, or more accurately, water retention. For example, if your body's responding to an allergy or intolerance, it will often retain water. So, when fasting, there's often a "quick-win" water loss that equates to an extra kilo being lost.

Q   What about fiber?

A   The process of juicing extracts the pulp (fiber) of the fruits and vegetables so on a juice fast it's a good idea to restore some bulk to maintain a healthy transit of waste matter through the gastrointestinal tract. Psyllium husks, a soluble form of fiber, do just the trick as, when taken with adequate amounts of fluids, they absorb water to form a large mass. In people with constipation, this mass stimulates the bowel to move, whereas in people with diarrhea it can slow things down and reduce bowel movements.

Some recent research also shows that psyllium husks may lower cholesterol. It's thought that the fiber stimulates the conversion of cholesterol into bile acid and increases bile acid excretion. In addition, psyllium husks may even decrease the intestinal absorption of cholesterol.

Psyllium comes from the plant Plantago ovata and is native to India. It is readily available in health food shops and online stores, either as husks or in powdered form. In non-fasting, normal dietary conditions, whole grains provide dietary fiber and similar beneficial effects to psyllium, so a supplement isn't needed unless recommended by your health care practitioner.

Q   Can colon cleansing help?

A   Your bowels are not just "poo pipes". Toxins and metabolic wastes from the blood and tissues are discharged into the intestinal canal to be excreted from the body. Not surprisingly, one of the long-established techniques to support the body's elimination organs during a fast is colon hydrotherapy or enemas. This is a technique that involves taking in water into the large intestine, also known as the bowel, to assist the removal of waste.

Colon hydrotherapy is not a new procedure. Enemas and rituals involving the washing of the colon with water have been used since pagan times. The first recorded mention of colon cleansing is on an Egyptian medical papyrus dated as early as 1500BCE. Ancient and modern tribes in the Amazon, Central Africa and remote parts of Asia have used river water for bowel cleansing, usually as part of magic-medical rites of passage performed by priests or shamans. Colon-cleansing therapies were an important part of Taoist training regimens and these therapies still form one of the fundamental practices of yoga teaching. Hippocrates, Galen and Paracelsus, who are recognized as the founding fathers of Western medicine, described, practiced and prescribed the use of enemas for colon cleansing. In Europe and the USA, colon-cleansing treatments were popular in the early decades of the 20th century and were often performed on patients by doctors practicing in sanatoria (health spas) and hospitals. From the 1920s to the 1960s, most medical practitioners were in favor of regular enemas, and these were often used as part of hospital treatment.

PART 3

REJUVENATION

FASTING AND MOTIVATION

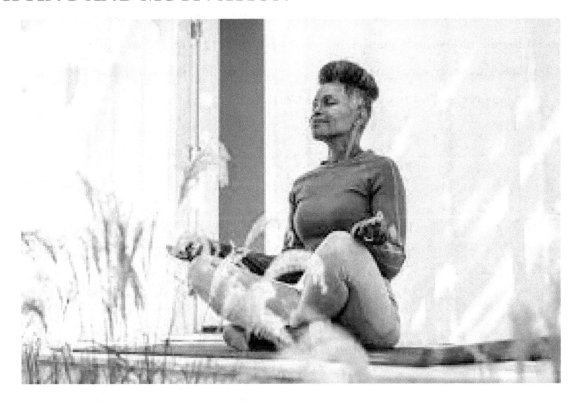

The final motivator, when thinking about incorporating fasting with exercise, is that it could give you more energy to train. There are lots of arguments over whether diet or exercise is more important when it comes to losing weight.

You may be familiar with the saying "you can't out-train a bad diet". While it's probably true that exercise alone isn't going to get you the body you want if you pay no attention to what you eat, dieting without exercise isn't a good idea either. After all, exercise comes with an impressive array of health benefits itself from heart and lung health, to stress relief, to maintaining strong bones.

When it comes to muscle strength and the way you look, exercise is the clear winner over diet. Researchers at Ann Arbor University in Michigan looked at how women's bodies responded to diet alone versus exercise alone. They found that, as expected, diet was more effective at reducing body weight, but exercise was more effective when it came to losing fat and maintaining muscle.

The thing is, getting the motivation to exercise can be hard when you're "on a diet" because you're always eating less than you're burning off and you often feel like you just don't have the energy. The good thing about fasting is that the gaps between meals are longer so when you do eat, you get to eat more. This means that you can time your exercise around the times when you've eaten and are feeling energetic. You're more likely to work harder!

MEDITATION

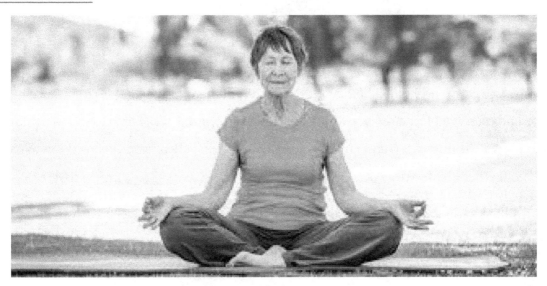

For those with ambition above and beyond the physical benefits of fasting, getting into the fasting state of mind can be helped by meditation, and if you have the time and inclination at least once in your life, a week's retreat can take the fasting experience to another level.

Meditation can be viewed in scientific terms for its effects on the mind and the body. During meditation, a marked increase in blood flow slows heart rate, and high blood pressure drops to within normal ranges. Recent research indicates that meditation can also boost the immune system and reduce free radicals – in effect, a slowing down of the ageing process.

There's much talk about the power of meditation and how you can use your mind to manifest great piles of money. But, becoming more aware of your mind is not just about manipulating it or attempting only to have positive thoughts – rather, it's about the ability to direct your attention toward or away from the mind at will.

My most intensive fast was on a 10-day silent meditation retreat during my time in India. One evening, five days into the experience when I was seriously doubting my judgement about freezing my butt off in a cold cave in the Himalayas, I had what I've come to realize was a "breakthrough" moment. In spiritual terms I'd describe it as a moment of grace. With a raw, pure energy of infinite magnitude, my mind flashed through formative experiences – good and bad – that had shaped my life. As my mind was swept along on this emotional rollercoaster, my body conveniently left the room, leaving me nowhere to run or hide… or at least that was how it felt!

Even more strangely (and I realize I may lose a few of you here!), during this experience it felt like my spine had dissolved to be replaced by a light-filled serpent. I was left astounded, uplifted and more than a little confused. Given that I was in the middle of a silent retreat, I couldn't even talk to anyone about what I had experienced.

It felt like all the vertebrae in my spine had dissolved at once, to be replaced with an energy much like an electric current. Even more bizarre was the fact that this energy surge was joined by an unshakable vision of a cobra-like snake replacing my spinal column.

Seeking answers, the day I left the meditation retreat I went straight to an Internet café. Within a few minutes I'd discovered that Hindu mythology describes the "serpent power" that lies coiled at the base of the spine as a kind of universal energy. Reportedly, this energy is awakened in deep meditation or enlightenment.

However, let me offer a word of caution before your expectations are set on a one-way ticket to nirvana. If, like many of us, you're the kind of person who never switches off, who even on holiday has the day scheduled from dawn till dusk, the mind experience that can accompany fasting may pass you by altogether. If you want to know yourself better, fasting in a gentle, supportive and quiet environment can help you accomplish a gentle re-boot both physically and mentally, and possibly a little spiritually too. Fasting needs some willpower in the beginning and patience as you move forward. Creating the right environment to enter the fasting state of mind, both inside and outside the body, is really helpful.

When I first started to meditate, I tried too hard. Furiously studying the science of the mind or contorting your face into Zen-like expressions won't work. The only way to experience meditation is actually to experience it. It can be maddening. You'll be trying to meditate for hours and then, just when you're ready to give up, you might get a flash of something akin to what you were aiming for. Yet, in that momentary shift you might see how you could choose to do a few things differently, or how some really small things have a huge impact on you, and how easy it would be to make a few minor changes. Many great thinkers have talked about breakthroughs and inspiration. The most famous of all was probably Albert Einstein, who said that no problem can be solved from the same level of consciousness that created it.

So, if you do manage to get your mind to stop its usual chatter through meditation, try asking yourself a question when all is calm. For example, if you always react to something uncomfortable by quashing the emotion with food, then meditation can create a gap to ask why. Sometimes there's a clear answer to that question, and sometimes there isn't. Usually, it takes a bit of time.

YOGA

Yoga is often lumped together with meditation since the kind of person who likes yoga is often into meditation, and vice versa. For people with a poor attention span, yoga can be a good way of getting into a calm state without the need ever to sit cross-legged.

There are many forms of yoga and it's a case of having a go and seeing which suits you best. Regardless of which tradition you choose, good yoga teachers can make you walk out of the class feeling a foot taller and ready to take on the world. My advice would be:

•   If you're gentle by nature, try Hatha.

•   If you're into precision and detail, go for Iyengar.

•   If you like the spiritual side of yoga, opt for Sivananda.

•   If you want yoga to help you sleep, try Yin.

•   If you're fit and physical, Ashtanga or Vinyasa "flow" yoga will be more your bag.

•   If you really want to sweat, try Bikram, or "hot yoga". It's not for the faint hearted and has some medical contra-indications, but it's considered seriously addictive by devotees.

SELF-CONTROL

If you're into popular psychology or consider yourself a "Tiger Mum" (or Dad), you might well have come across the famous longitudinal "Stanford University Marshmallow Study", first started in the 1960s by Stanford psychology researcher Michael Mischel. The purpose of the original experiment was to find out at what age children develop the ability to wait for something they really want, and subsequent studies over many years tracked the effects of deferred gratification on a person's future success. Mischel's experiment went like this:

NUTRITIONAL RULES FOR FASTING

EAT WELL

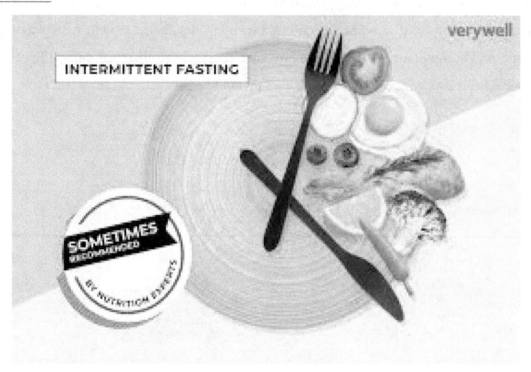

The problem with most fasting information is that it only focuses on the fasting bit, not on what you need to eat. If you're eating fewer calories, what you do eat becomes even more important. Why? We need nutrients for the glands and organs of the body to thrive and burn fat. Restricting nutrients by living on processed foods can deprive the body of the essential vitamins, minerals, fats and proteins it needs to maintain a healthy immune system, recover from injury or illness, keep muscles strong and maintain the metabolism. That's why this book includes these nutrition rules and practical fasting plans and recipes to help guide you.

RULE 1: ONLY EAT "REAL" FOOD

This means no fake food and no diet-drinks. If you grew up in the UK, chances are you'll have fond memories of bright orange corn snacks and fizzy drinks that turned your tongue red or blue. It's to be hoped that now you're "all grown up 'n' stuff", you eat lots of rocket and Parmesan salads, roasted artichoke and monkfish. If only that was the case for all of us. Celebrity chefs may make out that this is the norm but it just isn't. Most people still eat a diet full of processed, refined, low-fiber, nutrient-deficient foods.

Not all processed food is bad, though. In fact, some of it's great. Canned food without added sugar or salt and freshly-frozen fruit and veg are just a couple of examples of stellar staples for your larder. It's the low-calorie, low-fat, oh-so-easy snacks and meals that you need to watch out for since they're often loaded with chemicals and hidden sugars.

In many low-fat products the fat is simply replaced by processed carbohydrates in the form of sugar. Read the label of your regular low-fat treats (apart from dairy products where low fat is fine) and I'll bet you'll see words ending with "-ose". Various forms of sugar, be it sucrose, maltose, glucose, fructose, or the vaguely healthy-sounding corn syrup, are all bad news for weight gain, especially around the middle.

Heavily processed foods can also be high in chemicals. There's a real and present danger that chemicals in the environment may have a blocking effect on hormones that control weight loss. When the brain is affected by toxins, it's possible that hormone signaling is impaired. The reason why we're unsure as to the extent of the problem is that it's impossible to test for the thousands of chemicals that are contributing to the "cocktail" effect on the body. Err on the side of caution and control what you can. Keep foods "real"!

But what makes up a real-food diet?

PROTEIN

Protein is made up of amino acids, often called the "building blocks of life", and we need all of them to stay alive and thrive. Proteins from animal sources – meat, dairy, fish and eggs – contain all the amino acids and are therefore classed as "complete" proteins. Soya beans also fall into this category. Once and for all, eggs are healthy. Eggs have had a tough time of it over the years. First the salmonella scare, then the unfair link to cholesterol. Eggs are low in saturated fat and if you eat eggs in the morning, you're less likely to feel hungry later in the day.

Vegetable sources provide incomplete proteins. If you're vegetarian or vegan, you'll get your protein from nuts, seeds, legumes and grains but you need a good variety of these to ensure that you get the full range of essential amino acids.

TOP TIP:

•   Include more beans and lentils in your meals. Examples include kidney beans, butter beans, chickpeas or red and green lentils. They're rich in protein and contain complex carbohydrates, which provide slow and sustained energy release. They also contain fiber, which may help to control your blood fats. Try adding them to stews, casseroles, soups and salads.

CARBOHYDRATES

Carbs are one of the most controversial topics in nutrition and weight loss. For years we've been told that we eat too much fat, and that saturated fat is the main cause of heart disease. But recently, some experts have challenged this view, suggesting that carbohydrate is responsible for the obesity epidemic and a whole host of diseases. Should we cut carbs, avoid fat or simply reduce our food intake and exercise more?

When the body is starved of carbohydrates it looks for energy in its glycogen stores. Water binds to every gram of glycogen so it's easy to get dramatic weight loss – the only problem is that it's mostly water weight! Along with those glycogen stores you'll begin to lose fat but not at a rate higher than a healthier (and easier) weight-loss method.

The truth is there are healthy fats and healthy carbohydrates. Avoiding carbs altogether is unnecessary and potentially dangerous. The key is in recognizing that not all carbs are created equal. Low glycemic index (GI) carbohydrates, found in fiber-rich fruits, beans, unrefined grains and vegetables, are important for good health and can actively support weight loss – for example, through reducing appetite and energy intake.

However, high-GI refined carbohydrates, such as those found in soft drinks, white bread, pastries, certain breakfast cereals and sweeteners, not only make it harder to lose weight but could damage long-term health. Studies show that eating a lot of high-GI carbohydrates can increase the risk of heart disease and Type-2 diabetes.

TOP TIP:

• Eat bulky carbs to become slim. When you choose "big" foods like fruits, vegetables, salads and soups, which are bulked up by fiber and water, you're eating a lot of food that fills you up, but not a lot of calories.

FAT

Since fat is the greatest source of calories, eating less of it can help you to lose weight. However, fat is actually a vital nutrient and is an important part of your diet because it supplies the essential fatty acids needed for vitamin absorption, healthy skin, growth and the regulation of bodily functions. In fact, eating too little fat can actually cause a number of health problems.

The right kinds of fat, in the right amounts, can also help you to feel fuller for longer, so try not to think of fat as your mortal diet enemy, but rather a useful ally in the pursuit of your healthier lifestyle! Adding a little fat to your meals helps your body absorb nutrients and enhances the flavor of your food, so recipes have been created with this in mind. Choose monounsaturated fats or oils (e.g., olive oil and rapeseed oil) as these types of fats are better for your heart. Coconut oil can be a good choice for cooking as it's heat-stable.

TOP TIPS:

• Increase essential fats – aim for at least two portions of oily fish a week. Examples include mackerel, sardines, salmon and pilchards. Oily fish contains a type of polyunsaturated fat called omega 3, which helps protect against heart disease. If you don't eat fish, use flaxseed oil in salad dressing and snack on walnuts.

- If you use butter, stick to a thin scraping on bread and just a smidgen for flavor in cooking.

- Choose lean meat and fish as low-fat alternatives to fatty meats.

- Choose lower-fat dairy foods such as skimmed or semi-skimmed milk and reduced-fat natural yogurt.

- Grill, poach, steam or oven bake instead of frying or cooking with oil or other fats.

- Watch out for creamy sauces and dressings – swap them for tomato-based sauces. Add herbs, lemon, spices and garlic to reduced-fat meals to boost flavor.

- Use cheese as a topping, not a meal – in other words, no macaroni cheese! Choose cheese with a strong flavor, such as Parmesan or goat's cheese so that you only need to use a small amount.

RULE 2: CUT OUT SUGAR

Too much sugar makes you fat and has an ageing effect on the skin. Sugar links with collagen and elastin and reduces the elasticity of the skin, making you look older than your years. The recipes I provide use low-sugar fruits to add a little sweetness – and the occasional drizzle of a natural sweetener such as honey is fine – but, in general, sugar is bad news and best avoided.

TOP TIP:

• Stick to dark chocolate if you need a chocolate "fix" (which simply is the case sometimes!), as most people need less of it to feel satisfied.

RULE 3: WATCH THE ALCOHOL

Over the years the alcohol content of most drinks has gone up. A drink can now have more units than you think. A small glass of wine (175ml/5½fl   cup) could be as much as two units. Remember, alcohol contains empty calories so think about cutting back further if you're trying to lose weight. That's a maximum of two units of alcohol per day for a woman and three units per day for a man. For example, a single pub measure (25ml/¾fl oz) of spirit is about one unit, and a half pint of lager, ale, bitter or cider is one to one-and-a-half units.

TOP TIP:

• If you're out for the evening, try out some healthy soft drinks such as tonic with cordial, or an alcohol-free grape juice as a tasty substitute to wine. Alcohol-free beers are also becoming increasingly popular and are available in most pubs and bars.

RULE 4: EAT FRUIT, DON'T DRINK IT

If you consume around 1 liter (35fl oz/4 cups) fruit juice, remember you'll be imbibing 500 calories. That's fine if you're juice fasting, but too much if it's simply a snack. You could tuck into a baked potato with tuna and two pieces of fruit for the same number of calories.

TOP TIPS:

- Choose herbal teas (especially green tea, which may aid fat loss).

- Feel free to have a cup or two of tea or coffee. A small amount of milk is allowed but keep it to a splash when you're fasting.

- Sip water throughout the fast, aiming for a fluid intake of around 1.2–2 liters (40–70fl oz/4¾–8 cups) a day. This will not only help to keep hunger pangs at bay, it will also keep you hydrated.

RULE 5: AVOID THE PITFALLS

TOP TIPS:

• Top up before you fast. When you first start fasting, you may feel hungry during the times when you'd normally have a meal and you may also feel slightly light-headed if you have sugary foods as your last meal. This isn't a sign that you're wasting away or entering starvation mode, and these feelings of hunger will usually subside once that usual meal time has passed. Try to get your carbohydrate intake from fruit, vegetables and whole grains and eat a good amount of protein, which will fill you up for longer. Following the fasting plans will make this as straightforward as possible.

• Stock up for quick meals. Make sure you always have ingredients in your fridge and cupboards for meals that can be put together quickly, such as stir- fries, soups and salads.

• Don't polish off the kids' plates. Eating the children's leftovers is a fast track to weight gain for parents. Put the plates straight into the sink or dishwasher when the children have finished their meal, so you won't be tempted!

• Downsize your dinner plate. Much of our hunger and satiation is psychological. If we see a huge plate only half full, we'll feel like we haven't eaten enough. But if the plate is small but completely filled, we'll subconsciously feel that we have eaten enough.

• Beware of the Frappuccino effect. Black coffee only contains about 10 calories but a milky coffee can contain anything from 100 calories for a standard small cappuccino to a whopping 350+ calories for a Grande with all the trimmings. Much like the plate size, shrink your cup size and shrink your waist line. Don't be afraid to ask for half the milk – spell it out: "Don't fill up the cup." I do it all the time and the best baristas get it right first time!

• The sandwich has become the ubiquitous carb-laden "lunch on the go". Lose the top piece of bread to cut your refined carbohydrates and instead fill up with a small bag of green salad leaves and healthy dressing.

•　　Don't try to change everything at once. Bad habits are hard enough to break as it is. Focus on breaking one at a time.

•　　If you're a parent, choose your meal skipping wisely. I've tried fasting with a toddler who doesn't understand why Mummy isn't eating and will, quite literally, shove a fistful of tuna pasta into my mouth.

•　　Get the portions right. If you're restricting the number of meals you're having, it makes sense that the portion sizes need to be bigger than they would be if you were eating five mini-meals a day. Use the recipe section as a guide to how big your portions should be.

PART 4

ANTI-AGING EXERCISES

FITNESS RULES FOR FASTING

WHY EXERCISE?

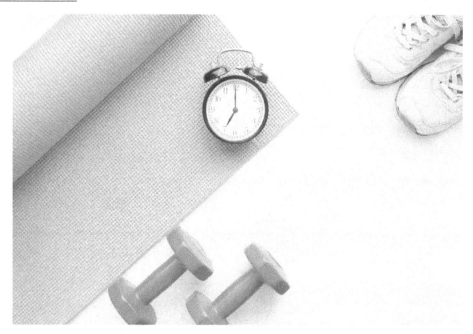

That old adage, "Daily exercise maketh for a healthy life and lively mind", is all well and good, but the saboteurs of all good intentions, Temptation, Procrastination and Distraction, tend to make exercise an erratic achievement for most people.

Exercise is especially challenging if you're juggling the demands of parenthood. Even though I know I'll feel much better afterwards, some days if my husband didn't proverbially kick me out of the door with my running togs on, I myself would most likely fall victim to the three scourges. Whether it's the long-drawn-out bedtime rituals of frisky toddlers or the clearing up of spaghetti-smeared kitchen walls, parenting saps desire to do anything at all in the evening other than collapse on the sofa with a glass of wine in hand to watch the latest Scandinavian import TV series. Or maybe that's just me.

But really, do we have to exercise? It's a question I'm often asked on retreat. Many people think that exercise is just about burning off calories, but there's so much more to it than that. Along with helping you to achieve and maintain your ideal weight, physical activity can do the following:

- Reduce your risk of heart disease, stroke, type-2 diabetes and some cancers.

- Help keep your bones strong and healthy.

- Improve your mood, reduce feelings of stress and help you sleep better.

- Give you strength and flexibility – attributes that seem to translate as much mentally as they do physically.

I also believe that on top of all these worthy benefits, exercise adds life to your years.

Sometimes it's a simple matter of making exercise more important to you. Also, if you're paying up front for an exercise class, you may find it's harder to miss. My days are dramatically improved by 30–60 minutes of exercise, whether it's running with my dog on the beach or Pilates with the girls. Exercise provides variety, buzz, a glow, a sense of achievement and perspective, plus it helps offset any guilt about enjoying that glass of Sauvignon at the end of the day!

HOW MUCH EXERCISE DO YOU NEED?

In 2010 the World Health Organization (WHO) issued global recommendations on the amount of physical activity we need to stay healthy. They recommend that adults (aged 18–64) should build up to at least 2½ hours of moderate intensity aerobic activity, 1¼ hours of vigorous intensity activity, or a combination of the two each week. We should also incorporate two sessions of muscle-strengthening activities, such as weight training, every week. Although we can meet these recommendations by doing just five 30-minute workouts a week, less than a third of British women are active enough for health. And the benefits don't stop at 30 minutes. WHO stresses that additional benefits can be achieved if we double these minimum recommendations.

Focus is often placed on structured physical activity, such as hitting the treadmill or a spin class, but this is far from being the only factor when it comes to the calorie-burn equation. We've all heard the advice about getting off the bus a stop early, or taking the stairs instead of the lift, but in reality, how useful is this? Well, just think about it… as technology progresses we're at our computers for longer and longer periods each day, we shop online rather than going to the high street, we catch up with friends over Skype or Facebook rather than meeting them in the flesh, we watch TV to relax at the end of a busy day and sometimes we're just so busy that we don't think we can allow ourselves an extra five minutes to walk rather than take the car… the thing is, if you're looking to lose weight, the total energy you burn off has to be higher than the amount you eat and every little step helps.

Collectively, unstructured activities are referred to as non-exercise activity thermogenesis (NEAT) and include all activity-related energy expenditure that's not purposeful exercise. NEAT is actually pretty cool since some of us actually alter NEAT levels according to what we eat without even thinking about it. In other words, one of the secrets of the naturally slim is that they fidget and move more if they over-eat. In fact, one of the ways I was taught to help identify different body types during my training in India was to notice how much of a fidget people were when I was consulting with them! Without fail, those who had "ants in their pants" were the naturally slender types. So, if you're more of a couch potato, walking off dinner is clearly a very good idea! A basic pedometer can track how far you walk each day, and trying to

beat yesterday's step count can be addictive. The next generation of activity monitors track every move you make, and some even help you to understand your sleep patterns.

WHAT COUNTS AS EXERCISE?

Physical activity doesn't just mean sweating it out at the gym – any movement that gets you slightly out of breath, feeling warm and a little bit sweaty, and that makes your heart beat faster, counts (yes, I know what you're thinking and that kind of workout counts too). You can choose from sport, active travel, structured exercise or housework. Even small changes are beneficial and you'll get more benefit from a brisk walk every day than from dusting off your gym membership card once a month. If you've never been very active, it's not too late to start. The key to developing an active lifestyle that you can keep up long term is to find an activity you enjoy.

FINDING INSPIRATION

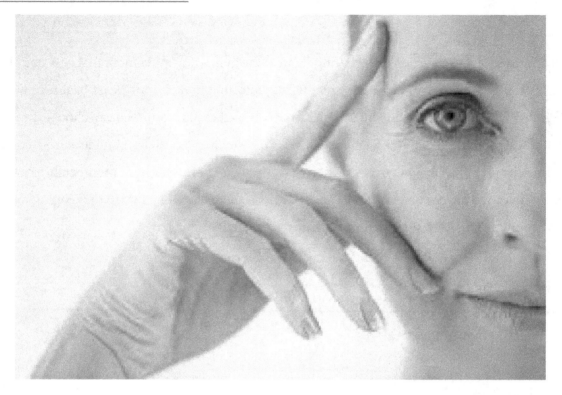

I've found that nothing works better than a bit of inspiration when it comes to changing habits. Over the last two decades, charity events such as marathons, 10km runs, cycle sportive and adventure racing have helped to motivate people to train with a goal in mind. Who would have thought that tens of thousands of women wearing sparkly bras would happily do the "Moonwalk" through the night in London and Edinburgh, kept going only by a sense of camaraderie and a shared purpose to raise money for breast cancer research?

Gyms, too, have revolutionized – it's no longer just about feeling the burn. Classes such as Zumba®, salsa and hula hooping, where having a laugh is every bit as important as burning off calories, have become part of many people's fitness regimes. "Outdoor gyms", like those run by military fitness types, have got all shapes, sizes and ages into the mud and pushing out the press-ups of a Sunday morning. For those willing to go even further, road-or mountain-biking, kitesurfing and triathlon provide accessible competitive events that you can now do much more easily at your own level.

TOP TIPS:

- Book an active holiday to get yourself started.

- Sign up for a charity run or hike.

- Achieve inner calm with yoga or sweat it out in a Bikram studio.

- If dancing's your thing, try Sh'Bam™, the latest craze to follow Zumba®.

- If you have kids, encourage them to play active games and join in too.

- Work off job frustrations with a boxing or martial arts class.

- Treat yourself to a one-to-one with a personal trainer.

- Volunteer for a local conservation project or do some heavy-duty gardening.

- Get back to what you were good at in school – badminton and netball are popular team sports that stand the test of time.

- Improve your commute to work by walking or cycling.

SIMPLE RULES FOR EXERCISE

RULE 1: TAKE THE FIRST STEP

As the saying goes, "Every journey starts with a single step". If there's anything preventing you from taking that first step, take some time to think about how you can overcome this. From there, set yourself a realistic activity goal for the week. Make sure you write it down and, even better, tell a loved one that you're thinking/going to do it – it makes it more real to share your conviction.

RULE 2: TAKE IT FURTHER

The next step is to monitor your progress – an activity diary is an ideal way to do this – and plan to add a little more each week. Keep setting new goals and challenging yourself. Variety is also vital as you can get into a rut with your exercise program just like with anything else. Follow the lead of international sport coaches who insist on variety to keep minds fresh and stimulated, or sign up to a sport where you'll be under the watchful gaze of a coach.

RULE 3: TAKE CARE

If you're new to exercise, or haven't done any for some time, you should always check with your doctor before starting a new exercise program. The benefits of activity almost always outweigh the risks, but if you have a health

condition or are just starting out, your doctor will be able to advise on any activities that you should avoid or take extra care with.

RULE 4: GO FOR THE BURN

You'll get the best benefits from a structured exercise plan, especially if you do some of your training at a high intensity and include some weights. But if you're not quite ready for that, fitting extra movement into your day is a good way to get started. If you take the stairs instead of the lift, get off the bus or train one stop early and are generally more active without actually working out, you could lose at least 6kg (1st) in 12 months, so long as you don't eat more to compensate! If you're already exercising regularly, instead of just focusing on doing more exercise, take every opportunity to do things the active way.

When you're fasting, a great way to boost your calorie burn is to focus on increasing your NEAT. Together with the advice below on exercising, this will make sure you're doing everything you can to achieve the best shape possible.

ACTIVITY	TIME NEEDED (MINUTES)
1. Skipping	8
2. Jogging	12
3. Gardening (weeding)	14
4. Swimming (leisurely pace)	14
5. Cycling (light effort)	14
6. Scrubbing the floor (vigorous effort)	15
7. Vacuuming	18
8. Dancing	19
9. Playing with children	21
10. Walking the dog	24
11. Food shopping (at the supermarket)	28
12. Driving a car	32
13. Computer work	43

You might be disheartened when the running-or step-machine tells you you've burnt 87 calories when you've been sweating for at least 15 minutes. After all, it

doesn't even add up to a skinny cappuccino. Don't despair! You burn fat even after exercise because you primarily use carbohydrate fuel during the exercise, which takes time to replace, so in the meantime, your body burns fat for energy. In other words, your metabolism is raised for a little while after your workout.

EXERCISING AND FASTING

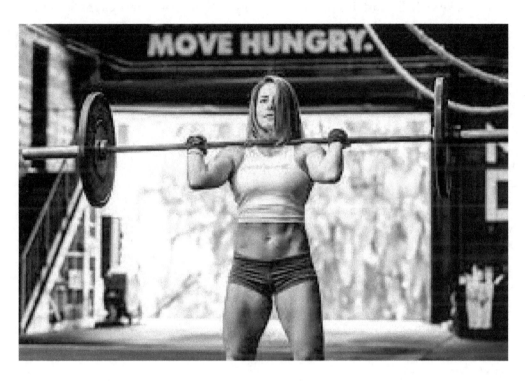

The obvious second part to the puzzle is exercise. Exercise has many wonderful benefits. It can help with depression and anxiety, while also helping you to attain your aesthetic goals. Exercise is also going to play a part in the balancing of the hormones mentioned earlier. Exercise promotes the production of HGH, but will also help drain glycogen stores quickly.

What is the best exercise when fasting?

It is popular belief that long drawn-out cardio at a steady pace is the best way to burn fat. In my experience, this is not the case. Although it has its benefits, when it comes to burning fat and the IF lifestyle, I've had far more success with HITT training for both female and male clients.

High Intensity Interval Training (HITT)

If burning fat is your mission, I recommend HITT training. Fast paced workouts that can be done in 30 minutes make this ideal for someone with a busy lifestyle. HITT can be done with bodyweight exercises, barbells, kettlebells and dumbbells. I usually look to use exercises that use more than one muscle group. For example, a row rather than a bicep curl. The name of the game is short bursts at near maximum effort. Below are some guidelines you can play with. They are meant as guidelines, not gospel!

- 20 second exercise – 10 second rest (Advanced)

- 10 second exercise – 20 second rest (Intermediate)

- 10 second exercise – 30 second rest (Beginner)

Rounds:

- 8+ (Advanced)

- 3-6 (Intermediate)

- 1-3 (Beginner)

Number of exercises:

- 7+ (Advanced)

- 5-6 (Intermediate)

- 3-5 (Beginner)

Example workouts

Beginner

- Squat

- Running on the spot

➢ Star Jumps

Intermediate

➢ Burpees

➢ Weighted squat

➢ Press Up

➢ Medicine Ball Slam

➢ Battle Ropes

Advanced

➢ Burpee/ High Jump

➢ Box Jump

➢ Kettlebell Swing

➢ Clean & Press

➢ Battle Ropes

➢ Kettlebell Row

EXERCISE AND THE 16/8 FAST

THE 16:8 DIET

	DAY 1	DAY 2	DAY 3	DAY 4	DAY 5	DAY 6	DAY 7
MIDNIGHT							
4 AM	FAST	FAST	FAST	FAST	FAST	FAST	FAST
8 AM							
12 PM	First meal	First meal	First meal	First meal	First meal	First meal	First meal
4 PM	Last meal by 8PM	Last meal by 8PM	Last meal by 8PM	Last meal by 8PM	Last meal by 8PM	Last meal by 8PM	Last meal by 8PM
8 PM	FAST	FAST	FAST	FAST	FAST	FAST	FAST
MIDNIGHT							

But what about exercising while fasting? As you'll know from the "Fit You and Your Life to Fasting" chapter, the 16/8 fasting pattern is often used by people who are looking to get into their best shape ever, and workouts are usually done in a fasted state.

However, it's important to remember that most of the studies on exercise while fasted were done on men, and we know that women's bodies may respond differently. This means that, when it comes to the 16/8 fast, the rules for men and women are slightly different.

EXERCISE AND THE 5/2 FAST

THE 5:2 DIET

DAY 1	DAY 2	DAY 3	DAY 4	DAY 5	DAY 6	DAY 7
Eats normally	Women: 500 calories Men: 600 calories	Eats normally	Eats normally	Women: 500 calories Men: 600 calories	Eats normally	Eats normally

If you're going to do the 5/2 fast, it's best to avoid prolonged or hard exercise on your 500-calorie days. However, it's fine to do this sort of exercise a couple of hours after your first meal the following day. And do make sure that if you're exercising the day before your 500-calorie day, you end the day with a proper meal.

Although you'll be going for periods of the day without food, the fasting plan covers all your nutritional requirements. To ensure that you're getting everything your body needs to fuel an active lifestyle, I encourage you to eat more during your eating "windows" if you feel hungry. Keep healthy snacks to hand so that you're not tempted by junk food if hunger pangs strike.

Recovery, Rest & The Importance of Sleep

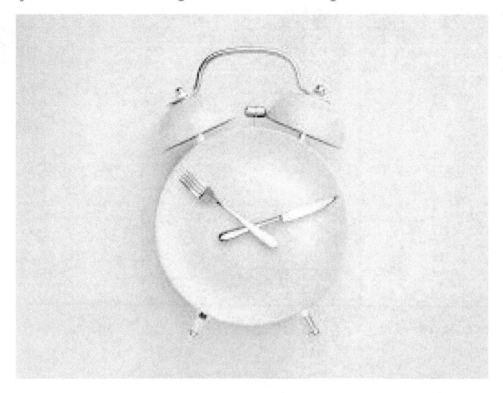

As promised, here is the third (perhaps most important) part of the weight loss puzzle which is often neglected. Sleep! Getting proper sleep can skyrocket your results - here's how.

Our body primarily enters an anabolic (building) type phase during sleep. Our body goes to work repairing damage, replacing cells, and believe it or not, burning fat. Shawn Stevenson explains this in his book "Sleep Smarter:

21 Essential Strategies to Sleep Your Way to A Better Body Better Health and Bigger Success". This book has outlined key hormones you should know about for weight loss, but there are many more. Some help initiate repair and growth and some help keep us awake and/or alert. One of the big factors dictating the creation and release of these hormones is quality sleep. Stevenson cites studies showing sleep deprivation can be linked to high levels of hormones such as cortisol and insulin (Remember what too much insulin does?). He also mentions hormones correlated with fat burning that are only secreted during sleep and darkness. Remember how HGH helps burn fat? Quality

sleep is linked to the creation of this hormone. If you're not getting quality sleep at the right times, all the exercise and healthy eating may not yield the results you were hoping for. If you've ever dieted before while thrashing yourself in the gym only to see little to no results, you know how frustrating this is! Perhaps proper sleep was the missing piece you needed!

4 tips to sleep better at night

TIP 1 – Get more sun

Our body's circadian system or "body clock" plays a huge role in the production of hormones. This is heavily influenced by sunlight. Stevenson explained Light, specifically morning sunlight, signals your glands and organs it's time to wake up, queuing them to produce day time hormones (most of these helping keep you alert and awake). If our bodies get inefficient sunlight in the morning and then too much artificial light at night (such as TV, laptops and smart phones) our circadian clock gets jumbled. This can cause our glands to produce hormones that prevent us sleeping. Lack of quality sleep is going to hinder the production of hormones such as HGH and could even spike the creation of hormones such as insulin. If this happens, we won't burn fat over night!

TIP2 – Avoid screens before bedtime

If you are someone who watches TV until 11pm or falls asleep to YouTube on your phone, the quickest way to improve sleep would be to stop using your devices at least an hour before bedtime. Remember how our body clock is impacted by sunlight? It's also impacted by artificial light. Our eyes are a major light sensor and the blue light produced by our favorite screens stimulate our body to produce day time hormones which are primarily for keeping us awake and active. With these bad boys circulating our body, falling asleep will be hard and our body won't produce those sweet anabolic hormones we need to repair and lose weight. Some of which Stevenson cited as only being produced in the dark. Interesting!

NOTE: My clients often argue that watching TV or some other device helps them go to sleep and without it they toss and turn. The information above is to achieve quality sleep and even though you might feel that way, I find in most cases this is simply because the client has made this a habit.

I encourage you to find other activities to replace your device, rather than lying in the dark stressing about not going to sleep.

TIP 3 – Sleep in darkness

Although this might seem apparent after the first two tips, some of my clients neglect this tip when not told. We can't control lights outside, such as street lamps and annoying security lights, but these could still affect our sleep on the molecular level, interrupting repair and leaving us tired the next day. Black out your windows with heavy duty curtains to stop pesky outside lights ruining your healing process!

P.S If it wasn't obvious turn out lamps, nightlights as well.

TIP 4 – Quality not Quantity

One of the most beneficial points I took away from Stevenson's book was that there is a sweet time window during the night where sleep is the most beneficial. During this window, our body produces the best number of hormones needed for repair and fat loss. He explained this was roughly between 10pm and 2am leaving every hour out of this window as a bonus. He also noted this could vary depending on time of year and what time zone you are in but suggested getting to bed as soon as possible after dark falls.

Improving your sleeping habits is key to weight loss, building muscle and living a healthier life in general. This important factor is often neglected in weight loss programs perhaps being the missing piece you needed! Quality sleep is going to ensure proper adaptation of key hormones for fat burning and might even be more important than increasing your exercise in the gym. Set a consistent bed time and make sure to get to bed about 30 to 60 minutes prior.

FASTING SAFELY

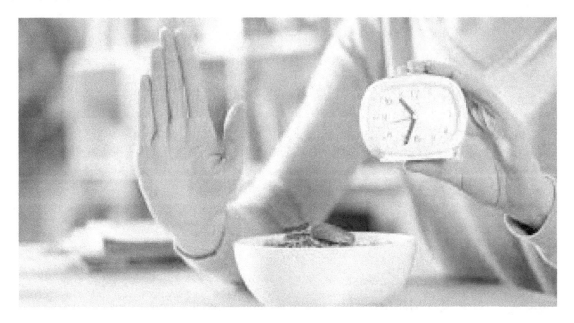

By now I hope that you have an open mind to the many benefits of fasting and that you're excited about giving it a go. If you've read this book and are still trying to decide if, when, or how to give fasting a try, remember that you'll only ever truly "get it" by trying it for yourself.

Before you launch headlong into your new fasting lifestyle, here are a few words of caution. Although fasting has been around for millennia, the science on how and when to fast is in its early stages. For example, there's very little research on how fasting affects fertility.

There are some people who should avoid fasting completely, some who should seek medical advice first, and some situations where it might not be right for you. Fasting isn't something that you should just jump into, and it doesn't suit everyone.

WHEN NOT TO FAST

You should avoid fasting if any of the following apply:

- You are pregnant, breastfeeding, or actively trying for a baby (it's okay to fast if you're getting your body ready to conceive, but please don't consider fasting if there's any chance you could already be pregnant).

- You have ever experienced an eating disorder.

- You are underweight

You should seek medical advice first if any of the following apply:

- You have a long-term medical condition such as cancer, diabetes, ulcerative colitis, epilepsy, anemia, liver, kidney or lung disease.

- You have a condition that affects your immune system.

- You are on medication, particularly medicines that control your blood sugar, blood pressure or blood lipids (cholesterol).

POSSIBLE SIDE-EFFECTS AND HOW TO MANAGE THEM

As we learnt earlier in the book, fasting may make you feel a bit "yucky" at first. Many juice fasters experience headaches through caffeine withdrawal, and feeling hungry is natural when you first try a fast. These effects don't usually last long, and most people find that they're outweighed by the positive effects of fasting.

More serious side-effects may include:

- Dehydration or over-hydration.

- Feeling dizzy or light-headed.

- Extreme fatigue.

- Constipation.

- Nausea or vomiting.

- Insomnia.

- Irregular periods.

Always err on the side of caution and stop the fast if you don't feel well. You can minimize the risk of some side-effects by approaching the fast safely.

END NOTE

I invite you to think of your goals as a journey. This book as the start, and your goal as the finish. The roads and paths in between will vary, and be full of both victories and losses. Your humble beginning and your eventual triumph mean nothing without the winding roads that link them, and vice versa. Everyone admires those who have "made it". Whether that is in regard to weight loss or some other human want like riches or fame. We are especially motivated by those who appear to have come from nothing or succeeded against all odds, but the road that links these two paradigms is just as important as the factors themselves. The roads are scarcely revered unless the end is reached, otherwise it is simply a road leading nowhere, a lost cause

– failure. Those who have nothing or are underprivileged are seldom celebrated unless they manage to follow a path with a successful ending. Your health and fitness journey are not exempt from such parameters. You have most likely started a hundred times. You have most likely trodden many paths seeking your goal, only to find fleeting success or failure. I hope this book will arm you with enough hope to start once again and lead you on the right path to your ultimate victory, perhaps inspiring those around you to take action and do the same.

Gourmet Keto Diet Cookbook
For Women After 50

By

Stacey Bell

Table of Contents

Introduction

If you're just a woman over 50 years of age, you may be much more involved in weight loss than you would have been at 30. Most women face a slower metabolism at this age at a rate of around 50 calories a day. A slower metabolism will make it incredibly difficult to control weight gain, along with reduced exercise, muscle degradation, and the propensity for increased hunger pangs. There are several diet options available to help lose weight, but the keto diet is amongst the most famous lately. The keto diet (or ketogenic diet, for short) is indeed a low-carb, high-fat diet that promises numerous health benefits. We have obtained several questions about keto's feasibility and how to adapt the diet in such a healthier way. More than 20 studies have shown that sort of diet can lead to weight loss and health enhancement. Diabetes, cancer, epilepsy, and Alzheimer's can still benefit from ketogenic diets. To make the body burn its very own fat stores more effectively, Keto is a diet that involves reducing carbohydrates and growing fats. Analysis has also shown that a keto diet is suitable for general health and weight reduction. In particular, ketogenic diets have enabled certain individuals to lose excess body fat without the extreme hunger pangs characteristic of most diets. Any patients with type 2 diabetes have also been shown to be able to use keto to manage their signs. At the core of a ketogenic diet are ketones. As an alternative energy source, the body creates ketones, a fuel molecule, while getting short on blood sugar. When you decrease carb consumption and eat only the proper levels of nutrients, ketone production happens. Your liver will convert body ketones when you consume keto-friendly foods, which are then used by your body as an energy supply. You are in ketosis as the body uses fat for energy supply. This causes the body, in some situations, to dramatically increase its fat burning, which helps to minimize pockets of excess fat. This fat-burning approach not only lets you lose some weight, but it could also fend off cravings during the day and eliminate sugar crashes. While it's straightforward to assume that the keto diet is high in fat and low in carbohydrates, while you're in the supermarket aisle, it still feels a little more complicated. If Keto is right for you or not depends on several variables. A ketogenic diet can have many advantages, especially for weight loss, providing you don't suffer from health problems. Eating a perfect mix of greens, lean beef, and unrefined carbohydrates are the most significant thing to note. It is possible that keeping the whole foods is the most successful way to eat healthily, mainly because it is a sustainable strategy. It is important to remember that a lot of literature suggests that it is impossible to continue with ketogenic diets. For this cause, discovering a safe eating plan that appeals to you is the right advice. It's cool to try good experiences, but don't leap headfirst. If you are a female over 50 and want to change your lifestyle, this book will teach you what you need to learn about the keto diet. Breakfast, lunch, dinner recipes, and some tasty keto snacks and smoothie recipes are tasty, convenient, and straightforward to make for you. To sustain a balanced lifestyle after 50, let's just begin reading.

Chapter 1: The Keto Diet: A Better Way Towards Improved Health for Women Over 50

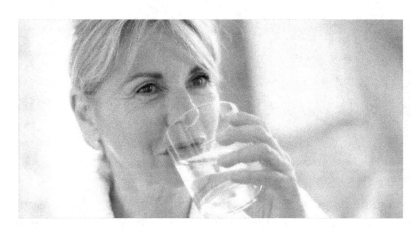

1.1. Keto diet in a nutshell

The keto diet is a high-fat, low-carbohydrate diet similar to Atkins & low-carb diets. It involves substantially reducing the consumption of carbohydrates and replacing them with fat. "Ketogenic" is a low-carb food idea (like the Atkins diet). The idea is to get more calories from proteins, fats, and less from carbohydrates. One has to remove carbohydrates such as starch, soda, pastry, and white bread, which are simple to digest. This reduction in calories takes the body to a regular cycle of the body, which is called ketosis. When this happens, the liver is extremely energy efficient when processing fat. It also transforms fat into ketones in the liver that can supply energy to the brain. Ketogenic diets can contribute to substantial decreases in blood sugar and insulin levels. This, combined with the increased ketones, has a range of health effects. If you eat less than 50 grams of carbohydrate a day, your body will eventually run out of fuel (sugar in your blood) and eat it easily. It normally takes about 3 and 4 days. Then you start to break down protein and energy fat that can help you drop weight. It's referred to as ketosis. It is necessary to note that the ketogenic diet is not about dietary benefits, but rather about a short-term diet that focuses on weight loss. People use ketogenic diets to lose weight most frequently, although they may also help to address certain medical problems, including epilepsy. People with heart disease, brain diseases, and even acne can benefit, but more research in these fields is required. First, talk to your doctor about whether a ketogenic diet is healthy, particularly if you have type 1 diabetes.

1.2. Yes, keto is fine for women over 50

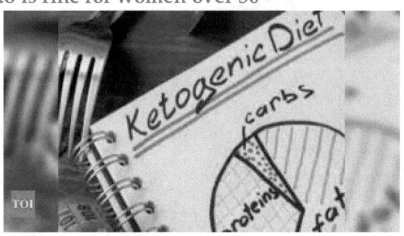

There are certain common dangers and issues that relate to anyone who consumes keto, such as the need to add electrolytes to prevent cramps. It's crucial for anyone to grasp the diet and do it appropriately. Especially for women above 50, it could mean paying particular attention to calcium or making sure they have enough food to remain well-nourished. There are still individuals – both men and women – who simply don't work on low-carb diets for a particular reason, and that's all right.

Some several unique concerns and subjects relate mainly or exclusively to women. Yet overall, there is very little proof that healthy women who are just not pregnant may be more worried about keto than some other diet. There is no proof that people necessarily cannot or cannot consume keto – in fact, there are many women who do keto and enjoy keto! And there is also some proof that keto diets can be beneficial to some female-specific problems, such as PCOS.'

1.3. Key takeaways for women above 50 on keto Diet

o   Get the correct protein quantity

o   Don't eat far too much fat.

o   fast intermittently

o   Look out for the creeping carb

o   Cut the alcohol out

o   Evite the sweeteners

o   Do a weightlifting workout

o   Get ample sleep right now

o   Reducing tension

o   Be rational about this

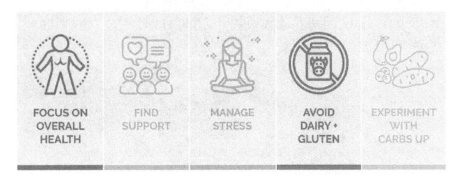

1.4. Problems to be aware of regarding keto diet in over 50 women

One issue that women can face with keto diets about the under-eating to the extent of a physically unsafe energy deficiency or a lack of body fat underneath a safe amount. It's quite likely to consume less on keto, deliberately or accidentally. Many people who pursue keto seem to be healthy-conscious individuals who want to exercise out a lot, which only increases the issue when they consume less, then drives themselves into intense exercises that need more protein and calories to recover.

This is much more harmful to women than for men since the female body is vulnerable to malnutrition. The reduction of bone mass, a higher likelihood of bone stress fractures, a higher risk of anemia, stomach issues, and psychiatric symptoms.

Dieting to the extent of missing your time can even happen without some workout at all, and it's almost as risky that way! Nutrition Disease

None of this is special to keto. It's all like the calorie deficit. But the appetizing benefits of keto diet increase the risks that women attempting to lose weight will not know how severe they are, mainly because they'll actually receive nothing but compliments about how "safe" they're eating and how "sweet" they're consuming absolutely nothing.

Although, of course, the repression of hunger often renders the diet appealing to women living with eating disorders. It's not exactly a "keto danger;" it's a danger of violating keto, but it does occur. It's outside the meaning of a single post to really consider coping with it, so it sounds like someone you meet, reach out to – you could be saving a life.

Chapter 2: Keto Breakfast recipes for women over 50

Let's be realistic; one of life's biggest pleasures is a carbohydrate-rich breakfast. There are plenty of safe and tasty keto-friendly breakfast meals. And there is a lot you're probably going to save them from trying someday.

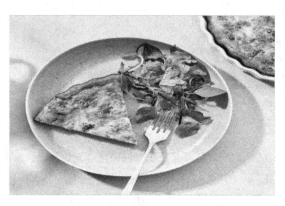

1. Keto Hot chocolate shake

Servings: 1 cup | Total time: 10 min

Calories: 193 | Proteins: 2g | Carbohydrates: 4 g | Fat: 18g

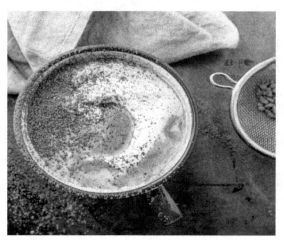

Ingredients

o   Two tablespoons unsweetened cocoa powder

o   Two and a half teaspoon sugar

o   One-fourth cup of water

o   One-fourth cup heavy cream

- o One-fourth teaspoon pure vanilla extract
- o Some whipped cream, for the purpose of serving

Steps of preparation

- o In a medium bowl on medium-low heat, mix together chocolate, swerve, and around two tablespoons of water until everything is smooth and absorbed. Increase down to

  a simmer, introduce remaining water & cream, and periodically whisk until heated.
- o Stir in the vanilla, and dump in the cup. Start serving with whipped cream or chocolate powder.

2. Keto delicious Cereal

Servings: 3 cups | Total time: 35 min

Calories: 188 | Proteins: 4g | Carbohydrates: 7 g | Fat: 17g

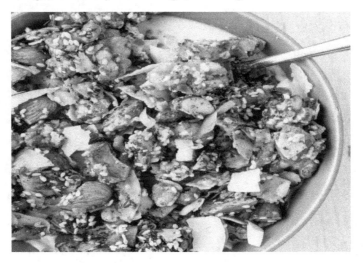

Ingredients

- o Cooking spray
- o One cup almond, chopped walnuts
- o One fourth cup sesame seeds
- o Coconut flakes
- o Two tablespoon flax seeds
- o Two tablespoon chia seeds
- o Half teaspoon ground clove
- o One and a half teaspoon ground cinnamon
- o One teaspoon pure vanilla extract

- o   Half teaspoon kosher salt
- o   One large egg white
- o   One-fourth cup melted coconut oil

Steps of preparation

- o   Preheat the oven to 350 ° C then oil the baking tray with a cooking spray. In a wide cup, add coconut flakes, almonds, sesame seeds, walnuts, and chia seeds and linseeds Stir with garlic, vanilla, salt, and cinnamon,
- o   Now Beat the egg white into foamy and mix in the granola. Apply the coconut oil and mix until all is well covered. Pour over the baking tray and scatter over a consistent layer. Bake for 20 mins just until it gets crispy, stirring gently halfway through. Let it just to cool completely.

3. Keto Sausage Sandwich

Servings: 3 | Total time: 15 min

Calories: 411 | Proteins: 38g | Carbohydrates: 7.3 g | Fat: 27g

Ingredients

- o   Six large eggs
- o   Two tablespoons heavy cream
- o   Pinch of red pepper flakes
- o   Pinch of Kosher salt
- o   Three slices cheddar
- o   Six frozen sausage patties
- o   Freshly ground black pepper
- o   One teaspoon butter
- o   Avocado in sliced pieces

Steps of preparation

- o   Beat the eggs, red pepper flakes, and heavy cream in a shallow cup. Season to taste with salt carefully. Melt the butter in a non - stick pan over medium heat. In the bowl, pour approximately 1/3 of the whites. Place the cheese mostly in center and then let it rest for around

1 minute. Place the corners of the egg in the center, shielding the cheese. Remove from heat and perform the same on remaining eggs.

o   Serve the eggs in two avocado sausage patties.

4. Ketogenic Cabbage Hash Browns

Servings: 2 | Total time: 10 min

Calories: 230 | Proteins: 8g | Carbohydrates: 6 g | Fat: 19g

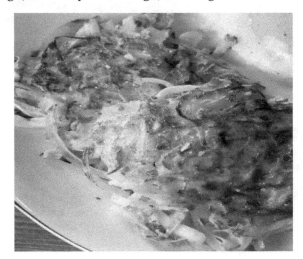

Ingredients

o   Two large eggs

o   Half teaspoon garlic powder

o   Half teaspoon kosher salt

o   Grounded black pepper

o   Two cups shredded cabbage

o   One fourth small yellow onion

o   One tablespoon vegetable oil

Steps of preparation

o   In a big cup, mix together eggs, salt and garlic. Season with salt and pepper. Apply the cabbage and the onion to the beaten egg and mix to blend.

o   Heat the oil skillet over medium-high flame. Roughly divide the prepared mixture into four patties in the skillet and pressure the spatula to compress. Cook until yellow golden and juicy.

5. Ketogenic Pancakes for breakfast

Servings: 6 | Total time: 15 min

Calories: 268 | Proteins: 9g | Carbohydrates: 6 g | Fat: 23g

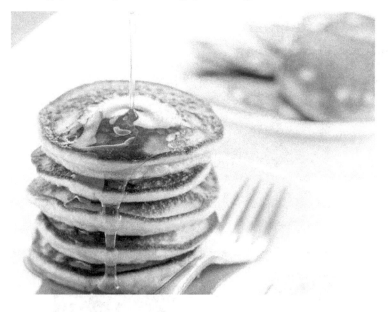

Ingredients

o   Half cup almond flour

o   Four oz. cream cheese

o   Four large eggs

o   One teaspoon lemon zest

o   Butter

Steps of preparation

o   In a medium cup, blend together the rice, the eggs, the cream cheese, and the lemon zest until soft and smooth.

o   Melt 1 tablespoon of butter on medium heat in a frying pan. Pour in approximately 3 teaspoons of the batter and simmer for 2 minutes until golden. Flip and cook for 2 more minutes. Move to the plate and continue for the remainder of the batter.

o   Serve with some sugar and butter.

6. Keto breakfast quick Smoothie

Servings: 6 | Total time: 5 min

Calories: 152 | Proteins: 1g | Carbohydrates: 5 g | Fat: 13g

Ingredients

o   One and a half cup frozen strawberries

o   One and a half cup frozen raspberries, plus more for garnish (optional)

o   One cup frozen blackberry

o   Two cup coconut milk

o   One cup baby spinach

o   Shaved coconut for garnishing purposes

Steps of preparation

o   Combine all the ingredients (except coconut) in a mixer. Mix so that it gets creamy.

o   Divide, if used, into cups and top with raspberries and coconut.

7. Keto Breakfast Cups

Servings: 12 cups | Total time: 40 min

Calories: 82 kcal | Proteins: 6g | Carbohydrates: 1 g | Fat: 2g

Ingredients

o   Two pounds ground pork

o   Two tablespoon freshly chopped thyme

o   Two cloves of minced garlic

o   Half teaspoon paprika

o   Half teaspoon. ground cumin

o   One teaspoon kosher salt

o   Half cup ground black pepper.

o   One cup chopped fresh spinach

o   White cheddar shredded

o   Twelve eggs

o   One tablespoon freshly chopped chive

Steps of preparation

o Start by preheating the oven to 400 ° F. Mix the ground pork, garlic, paprika, thyme, salt and the cumin in a large dish. Now season with a salt and the pepper.

o Add just that small handful of pork per muffin container, and then push the sides to create a cup. Start dividing spinach and cheese similarly in cups. Crack the egg at the top of every cup and add salt and pepper for seasoning.

8. Keto Breakfast Blueberry Muffins

Servings: 12 muffins | Total time: 40 min

Calories: 181 kcal | Proteins: 4.5g | Carbohydrates: 25 g | Fat: 5.6g

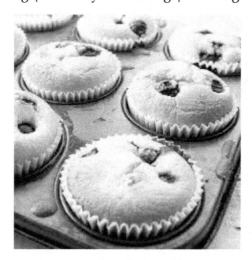

Ingredients

o Two and a half cup almond flour

o One third cup keto friendly sugar

o One and a half teaspoon baking powder

o Half teaspoon baking soda

o Half teaspoon kosher salt

o One-third cup melted butter

o One-third cup unsweetened almond milk

o Three large eggs

o One teaspoon pure vanilla extract

o Two-third cup blueberries

o Half lemon zests

Steps of preparation

o Start by preheating the oven to a temperature of 350 ° and put in a muffin tray with cupcake liners.

o In a big container, stir together almond flour, Swerve, baking soda, baking powder, and salt. Gently stir in melted butter, eggs, and vanilla once mixed.

o Gently fold the blueberries and the lemon zest until uniformly spread. Scoop equivalent quantities of the mixture into each liner of cupcakes and bake until softly golden and a toothpick inserted into the middle of the muffin comes out clean, this will happen within 23 minutes. Let it cool slightly before serving.

9. Keto Thai Beef Lettuce Wraps

Serving: 4 | Total Time: 30 min |

Calories: 368 Kcal, Fat: 14.5g, Net Carbs: 3.1g, Protein: 53.8g

Ingredients

o Olive oil 1 tablespoon

o Ground beef 1.5lb.

o Beef stock 1 ½ cups

o Garlic 2 cloves, minced

o lime juice fresh ¼ cup

o Fish sauce 2 tablespoons

o Chopped parsley ½ cup

o Mint chopped ½ cup

o To taste salt & pepper

Steps of Preparation

o Heat the olive oil over medium to high heat in a skillet.

o In a skillet, brown the beef for eight to ten mins.

o Add beef to skillet.

o Cook till the stock has fully boiled off.

o Meanwhile, mix the garlic, fish sauce, and lime juice.

o Add beef to the lime mixture.

- o Cook 2 to 3 mins.

- o Garnish with chopped herbs.

- o Assemble, the beef is scooped over the leaves of the cabbage or the lettuce.

- o Serve.

10. Breakfast **Skillet Cilantro-Lime Chicken**

Serving 4 | Total Time: 30 min

Calories: Kcal 426, Fat: 16.4g, Net Carbs: 6g, Protein: 61.8g

Ingredients

- o Olive oil 1 tbsp

- o Chicken breasts 4 boneless skinless

- o Kosher salt

- o Ground freshly black pepper

- o Unsalted butter 2 tbsp

- o Garlic minced 2 cloves

- o Medium limes 2 finely grated zest

- o Lime juice freshly squeezed 1/4 cup

- o Freshly chopped cilantro leaves & tender stems 1/3 cup

- o (Optional) for serving cooked rice

Steps of Preparation

- o Pat the chicken, thoroughly dry using paper towels. Season properly with pepper and salt. Steam 1 tbsp of the oil over medium to high shimmering steam in a ten-inch or bigger skillet. If possible, working in batches, add the chicken and sear to the bottom for 5 to 7 minutes, until deeply browned. Flip the meat, then sear for 5 to 7 mins before the other side is browned. Place the chicken into a plate; put aside.

- o Reduce to medium heat. Attach the garlic, butter, and lime zest then cook for 1 minute, stirring frequently. Stir in the juice of the lime. Send the chicken back to the skillet and any leftover juices. Cover, heat is reduced as required to maintain a moderate simmer and cook till the meat is cooked through and record 165°F on thermometer instant-read, 2 to 3 min.

- o Stir some of the sauce and the cilantro and pour over the chicken. When desired, eat with rice.

11. Breakfast keto Buffalo Chicken

Serving 4-6 | Total Time: 29 min

Calories: 295 Kcal, Fat: 12.6g, Net Carbs: 0g, Protein: 42.6g

Ingredients

o   Boneless chicken breasts 2 1/2 pounds skinless

o   Bottle hot sauce 1 (12-ounce)

o   Ghee or unsalted butter 4 tbsp

Steps of Preparation

o   In a 6-quarter or Electric Pressure Cooker, bigger Instant Pot put 2 1/2 pounds of chicken breasts boneless, skinless into one layer. Pour 1 (12-ounce) spicy chicken sauce bottle over it. Cube 4 tbsp of ghee or unsalted butter, then put the chicken on top.

o   Lock the cover in place and ensure that the valve is shut. High pressure cooking to cook about 15 minutes. It's going to take 10 - 12 minutes to work up under pressure. Once the time for cooking is finished, let the pressure drop for 5 min naturally. Release the remaining pressure

o   Move the chicken right away to a clean cutting plate. For slice the meat, using two forks, then move to a dish. Whisk the sauce once mixed and emulsified in a pressure cooker. Apply to chicken 1 cup sauce and flip to coat. Apply more sauce if appropriate and set aside any leftover sauce to consume or store.

12. Chocolate Breakfast Keto Protein Shake

Servings: 1 | Total time: 40 min

Calories: 445 kcal | Proteins: 31g | Carbohydrates: 7 g | Fat: 12g

Ingredients

o   Three fourth cup almond milk

o   Half cup ices

o   Two tablespoon almond butter

o   Two tablespoons unsweetened cocoa powder

o   Two tablespoons keto-friendly sugar

o   One tablespoon chia seed

- o Two tablespoon hemp seeds
- o Half table pure vanilla extract
- o A Pinch of kosher salt

Steps of preparation

- o Mix all ingredients together in a blender and process until smooth. Pour in a bowl and compote with a little more chia & hemp seeds.

13. Breakfast Bell Pepper Eggs

Servings: 3 yields | Total time: 20 min

Calories: 121 kcal | Proteins: 8.6g | Carbohydrates: 4 g | Fat: 7.9g

Ingredients

- o One bell pepper
- o Six eggs
- o Pinch kosher salt
- o Pinch of freshly ground black peppers
- o Two tablespoon chopped chives
- o Two tablespoon chopped parsley

Steps of preparation

- o Warm a nonstick saucepan over medium heat then gently oil with a cooking mist.
- o Place the bell pepper ring in the pan and simmer for 2 minutes. Swap the ring, then break the egg there in the middle of it. Add salt and pepper, then simmer until the egg is prepared to your preference for two to four minutes.
- o Repeat the same procedure with other eggs and serve with the chives and the parsley.

14. Omelet-Stuffed Peppers

Servings: 4 | Total time: 1 hour

Calories: 380 kcal | Proteins: 26g | Carbohydrates: 4.5 g | Fat: 28g

Ingredients

- o Two bell peppers
- o Eight eggs

o   One fourth cup milk

o   Four slices of bacon cooked

o   One cup shredded cheddar

o   Two tablespoon finely chopped chives

o   A pinch of Kosher salt

o   Black pepper crushed

Steps of preparation

o   Preheat the oven to 400 ° C. Now place the peppers sliced horizontally in a big baking sheet. Apply a very little water to the sheet and bake the pepper for five minutes.

o   In the meanwhile, beat the eggs and milk together. Stir in sausage, cheese, and chips and add salt and pepper as required.

o   When the peppers are baked, apply the egg mixture to the peppers. Place in the oven and cook for 35 to 40 minutes until the eggs have been set. Garnish with a little more chives and eat.

15. Keto breakfast Clouded Bread

Servings: 6 rolls | Total time: 35 min

Calories: 98 kcal | Proteins: 4g | Carbohydrates: 0.2 g | Fat: 9g

Ingredients

o   Three large eggs

o   One fourth teaspoon cream of tartar

o   A Pinch of kosher salt

o   Two oz. cream cheese

o   One tablespoon Italian seasoning

o   One tablespoon shredded mozzarella

o   Two teaspoon tomato paste

o   Pinch of kosher salt

o   One teaspoon poppy seed

o   One teaspoon sesame seed

o   One teaspoon minced dried garlic

o   One teaspoon minced dried onion

Steps of preparation

o Start by preheating the oven to 300 ° C and cover a wide pan with parchment paper.

o Separate the egg whites from its yolks in 2 small glass containers. Apply the cream of the tartar and the salt to the egg whites, then with a hand blender, beat until solid. It will happen within 2 to 3 minutes. Transfer the cream cheese to the egg yolks and now, using a hand blender, combine the yolks and the cream cheese until blended. Gently incorporate the egg yolk mixture in the egg whites.

o Divide the dough into portions of 8 mounds on a lined baking sheet, 4 "off from each other — Bake until it becomes golden, which will happen within twenty-five to thirty minutes.

o Instantly sprinkle each slice of bread with cheese and oven for two or three minutes. Let it cool a bit. Easy plain cloud bread is ready for you.

o Add 1 tablespoon of Italian seasoning, two tablespoons of shredded mozzarella or parmesan cheese, and two tablespoons of tomato paste to the egg yolk mixture. Add 1 tablespoon of Italian seasoning, two tablespoons of shredded mozzarella or parmesan cheese, and two tablespoons of tomato paste to the egg yolk mixture. Bake until it becomes golden, which will happen within twenty-five to thirty minutes.

o Add 1/8 teaspoon of kosher salt, 1 teaspoon of poppy seeds, 1 teaspoon of sesame seeds, 1 teaspoon of mashed dried garlic, then 1 teaspoon of chopped dried onion to the egg yolk mixture. (Or use 1 tablespoon with all bagel seasoning.) All bagel cloud bread is set.

o Add 1 1/2 teaspoons of ranch seasoning powder to the egg mixture. Bake until it becomes golden, which will happen within twenty-five to thirty minutes. Ranch cloud bread is ready to go.

16. Breakfast Jalapeño Popper Egg Cups

Servings: 12 cups | Total time: 1 hour

Calories: 157.2kcal | Proteins: 9.5 g | Carbohydrates: 1.3 g | Fat: 12.2 g

Ingredients

o Twelve slices bacon

o Ten large eggs

o One fourth cup sour cream

o   Half cup shredded Cheddar

o   Half cup shredded mozzarella

o   Two jalapeños, one minced and one thinly sliced

o   One teaspoon garlic powder

o   A pinch of kosher salt

o   Cooking spray

o   Ground black pepper

Steps of preparation

o   Preheat the oven to 375 ° C. Cook the bacon in a wide medium saucepan until it is well golden brown and still stackable. To drain, put aside on a paper towel-lined dish to drain.

o   In a large plastic container, stir together eggs, cheese, sour cream, jalapeno minced, and garlic powder. Season to taste with salt & pepper.

o   Use a nonstick cooking spray to oil the muffin tin. Fill each well along with one slice of bacon, then add the egg mixture into each muffin tin until around two-thirds of the way to the tin's top   Cover each muffin with a slice of jalapeno.

o   Bake for a period of 20 minutes just until the eggs are no longer sticky. Cool briefly before withdrawing the muffin tin.

17. Keto Zucchini Breakfast Egg Cups

Servings: 18 cups | Total time: 35 min

Calories: 17 kcal | Proteins: 1 g | Carbohydrates: 1.3 g | Fat: 1 g

Ingredients

o   Cooking spray

o   Two zucchinis peeled

o   One fourth lb. ham

o   Half cup cherry tomatoes

o   Eight eggs

o   Half cup heavy cream

o   A pinch of Kosher salt

o   A grounded black pepper

- o Half teaspoon dried oregano
- o One Pinch red pepper flakes
- o One cup shredded cheddar

Steps of preparation

- o Start by preheating the oven to 400 ° F and oil the muffin tray with a cooking mist. To form a crust, line inside and underside of muffin tin with both the zucchini strips. Sprinkle with the cherry tomatoes and the ham each crust.
- o In a medium container, stir together eggs, whipping cream, oregano & red pepper flakes and add salt and pepper. Pour the egg mixture over the ham and tomatoes and cover with the cheese.
- o Bake for 30 minutes until eggs are ready.

18. Breakfast Brussels Sprouts Hash

Servings: 4 cups | Total time: 40 min

Calories: 181 kcal | Proteins: 3 g | Carbohydrates: 13 g | Fat: 14 g

Ingredients

- o Six slices bacon
- o Half chopped onion
- o One lb. Brussels
- o An inch of Kosher salt
- o Black pepper grounded
- o One fourth teaspoon crushed red pepper flakes
- o Two minced cloves garlic
- o Four large eggs

Steps of preparation

- o Cook bacon until crispy in a large frying pan. Switch off the heat and move the bacon to a paper towel tray. Hold much of the bacon fat in the pan, cut some black specks from the pan.

o   Turn the heat down to low and transfer the onion and Brussels to the pan. Cook, stirring regularly before vegetables start to turn soft and turn golden. Season to taste with salt, pepper & red pepper flakes.

o   Transfer 2 tablespoons of water in the mixture and cover the pan. Cook till the Brussels are soft, and the water gets evaporated for about five minutes. (If all the water is gone until the sprouts are soft, add a little more water to the pan and cover for a few more minutes.) Put the garlic to the pan. Cook until fragrant for almost 1 minute.

o   Cut four holes in the hash using a wooden spoon, to expose the base of the pan. Break an egg into each gap and add salt and pepper for each egg. Replace the lid and cook it until eggs are ready to your taste, which is around 5 minutes for the egg that is runny

o   Sprinkle the cooked bacon bites over the whole pan and serve hot.

19. Best Breakfast Keto Bread

Servings: 1 bread | Total time: 40 min

Calories: 165 kcal | Proteins: 6 g | Carbohydrates: 3 g | Fat: 15 g

Ingredients

o   One fourth cup butter, melted and cooled

o   One and a half cup ground almond

o   Six large eggs

o   Half teaspoon cream of tartar

o   One tablespoon baking powder

o   Half teaspoon kosher salt

Steps of preparation

o   Start by preheating the oven to 375 ° F and then line the 8"-x-4 "loaf on a baking sheet. Completely separate egg whites from egg yolk.

o   In a wide container, mix egg whites with tarter cream. Using a hand blender, keep whipping until strong peaks are created.

o   Shake the yolks with melted butter, baking powder, almond flour, and salt in a separate big bowl using a hand blender. Fold in 1/3 of egg whites when completely blended, then fold in the remainder.

o Load the batter into the loaf pan and make flat layer. Then Bake for 30 minutes or until the surface is softly golden, and the toothpick comes out clean. Enable to cool for 30 minutes before cutting.

20. Bacon Breakfast Avocado Bombs

Servings: 4 bombs | Total time: 25 min

Calories: 251 kcal | Proteins: 6 g | Carbohydrates: 13 g | Fat: 18 g

Ingredients

o Two avocados

o One-third shredded Cheddar

o Eight slices bacon

Steps of preparation

o Steam the broiler and line up a narrow baking sheet with foil.

o Cut each avocado into half and scrape the pits. Take the skin off from each of the avocados.

o Cover two-thirds of the cheese, and substitute with the other thirds of the avocado. Cover 4 pieces of bacon in each avocado.

o Put the bacon-wrapped avocados upon this lined baking sheet and broil till the bacon is crisp, approximately 5 minutes. Turn the avocado really carefully and proceed to cook till crispy all around, approximately five minutes per side.

o Break half lengthwise and serve instantly.

21. Breakfast Ham & Cheese keto Egg Cups

Servings: 12 cups | Total time: 35 min

Calories: 108 kcal | Proteins: 10.4 g | Carbohydrates: 1.2 g | Fat: 5.9 g

Ingredients

o Cooking spray

o Twelve slices of ham

o One cup shredded cheddar

o Twelve large eggs

o A pinch of Kosher salt

- o Ground black pepper
- o Parsley, for garnish

Steps of preparation

- o Preheat the oven to 400o and oil the 12-cup muffin tray with a cooking mist. Top each cup with just a piece of ham and top with cheddar. Break an egg inside each ham cup and add salt and pepper.
- o Bake until the eggs are roasted thru, 12 to 15 minutes.
- o Garnish with parsley, serve.

22. Keto Breakfast Peanut Fat Bombs

Servings: 12 bombs | Total time: 1 hour 40 min

Calories: 247 kcal | Proteins: 3.6 g | Carbohydrates: 3.3 g | Fat: 24.4 g

Ingredients

- o Eight oz. cream cheese
- o A pinch of kosher salt
- o Half cup dark chocolate chips
- o Half cup peanut butter
- o One fourth cup coconut oil

Steps of preparation

- o Line a narrow baking sheet with a sheet of parchment paper. In a medium container, mix cream cheese with peanut butter, 1/4 cup of coconut oil, and some salt. Using a hand blender, beat the mixture until it becomes thoroughly mixed, approximately for 2 minutes. Put the bowl in the freezer until it is lightly firmed, for 10 to 15 minutes.
- o When a peanut butter mixture is formed, use a tiny cookie scoop to produce spoonful-sized balls. Put in the refrigerator for 5 minutes to harden.
- o In the meantime, produce a chocolate drizzle by mixing chocolate chips and the leftover coconut oil in a large mixing bowl and microwave it for 30 seconds until completely melted. Drizzle over the balls of peanut butter and then put in the refrigerator for 5 minutes.
- o Keep wrapped in the refrigerator to stock.

23. Breakfast keto Paleo Stacks

Servings: 3 | Total time: 30 min

Calories: 229 kcal | Proteins: 3 g | Carbohydrates: 11 g | Fat: 18 g

Ingredients

o   Three sausage patties

o   One mashed avocado

o   A pinch of kosher salt

o   Ground black pepper

o   Three large eggs

o   Hot sauce as required

Steps of preparation

o   Heat the breakfast sausage.

o   Mash the avocado onto the breakfast sausage and add salt and pepper.

o   Spray a medium pan over medium heat with only a cooking spray and then spray the interior of the mason jar cap. Place the mason jar lid within middle of the pan and break the egg inside. Add salt and pepper and cook for 3 minutes until hot, then remove the cover and continue to cook.

o   Place the egg on top of the mashed avocado. Season with chives and sleet with the hot sauce you want.

24. Breakfast keto quick chaffles

Servings: 2 yields | Total time: 25 min

Calories: 115 kcal | Proteins: 9 g | Carbohydrates: 1 g | Fat: 8 g

Ingredients

o   Four eggs

o   8 oz. shredded cheddar cheese

o   Two tablespoon chives

o   A pinch of salt and pepper

o 4 eggs for toppings

o Eight bacons

o Eight cherry tomatoes diced

o Two oz. baby spinach

Steps of preparation

o Organize the bacon slices in a big, unheated pan and set the temperature to moderate flame. Golden brown the bacon for 8-12 mins, turning often, until crispy to bite.

o Put aside on a paper towel to drain when you're cooking.

o Put all of the waffle ingredients in a mixing container and blend well.

o Lightly oil the waffle iron and afterward uniformly spoon the mixture over the bottom of the tray, spreading it out gently to achieve even outcomes.

o Shut the waffle iron and cook for roughly. 6 minutes, depending on capacity of the waffle maker.

o Crack an egg in the bacon fat in the cooking pan and cook slowly until finished.

o Serve each tablespoon of scrambled egg and bacon pieces along with some baby spinach and some sliced cherry tomatoes.

25. Keto breakfast with fried eggs, tomato, and cheese

Total Time: 15 mins | Serving 1

Calories: Kcal 417, Fat:33g, Net Carbs:4g Protein:25g

Ingredients

o Eggs 2

o Butter ½ tbsp

o Cubed cheddar cheese 2 oz

o Tomato ½

o Ground black pepper & salt

Steps of Preparation

o Heat butter over medium heat in a frying pan.

- o Season the diced side of the tomato with salt & pepper. Put the tomato in a frying pan.
- o Break the eggs in the same pan. Leaving the eggs to scramble on one side for eggs sunny side up. Rotate the eggs for a couple of mins and cook for one more minute for eggs fried over quickly. Cook for a few more minutes for tougher yolks. Season with salt & pepper.
- o On a plate, Put the eggs, tomatoes, and cheese to eat. Scatter with dried oregano eggs and tomatoes for some additional flavor and taste.

26. Keto eggs Benedict on avocado

Total Time: 15 mins | Serving 4

Calories: Kcal 522, Fat:48g, Net Carbs:3g Protein:16g

Ingredients

Hollandaise

- o Egg yolks 3
- o Lemon juice 1 tbsp
- o Salt & pepper
- o Unsalted butter 8½ tbsp

Eggs benedict

- o Pitted & skinned avocados 2
- o Eggs 4
- o Smoked salmon 5 oz

Steps of Preparation

- o Take a mason jar or other microwave-safe containers that will fit easily inside the immersion blender. Put the butter and then melt for around 20 seconds in the microwave.
- o In butter, incorporate the yolks of egg and lemon juice. The hand blender is Placed at the container bottom and combine until a creamy white coating is created. Raise the blender and lower it slowly to create a creamy sauce.
- o Place a saucepan over the stove with water and boil. Decrease the heat to low.

o Crack the eggs, one at a time, in a cup, and then carefully slip each into the bowl. Stirring the water in a circle can keep the egg white from displacing too much from the yolk. Cook 3-4 mins, depending on the yolk quality you like. To retain excess water, remove the eggs with a spoon.

o Break the avocados in two and remove the skin and stones. Create a slice of each half around the base, so it rests equally on the dish. Cover with one egg every half, then finish with a hollandaise sauce generous dollop. Load some smoked salmon.

o This dish must be consumed promptly and should not preserve or reheat. Hollandaise sauce Leftover can be preserved for up to 4 days in a fridge.

27. Keto quick low carb mozzarella chaffles

Total Time: 8 mins | Serving 4

Calories: Kcal 330, Fat:27g, Net Carbs:2g Protein:20g

Ingredients

o Melted butter 1 oz.

o Eggs 4

o Shredded mozzarella cheese 8 oz

o Almond flour 4 tbsp

Steps of Preparation

o Heat the waffle maker.

o Put all of the ingredients in a mixing bowl and beat to blend.

o Lightly oil the waffle iron with the butter, then spoon the mixture uniformly over the bottom, spreading it out to achieve an even outcome. Cover the waffle iron, then cook depending on the waffle maker, for approx. 6 mins.

o Release the cap softly when you feel it's done.

o Serve with favorite toppings.

28. Nut-free keto bread

Total Time: 50 mins | Serving 20

Calories: Kcal 105, Fat:8g, Net Carbs:1g Protein:6g

Ingredients

o Eggs 6

o Shredded cheese 12 oz

o Cream cheese 1 oz

o Husk powder ground psyllium 2 tbsp

o Baking powder 3 tsp

o Oat fiber ½ cup

o Salt ½ tsp

o Melted butter 1 tbsp

Topping

o Sesame seeds 3 tbsp

o Poppy seeds 2 tbsp

Steps of Preparation

o To 180 ° C (360 ° F), preheat the oven.

o Whisk eggs. Attach the cheese and the other ingredients, except the butter, and stir properly.

o Grease a buttered bread pan (8.5 " x 4.5 "x 2.75," non-stick or parchment-papered). Spread the dough with a spatula in the bread-pan.

o Sprinkle with poppy and sesame seeds over the rice. 35 Mins to bake the loaf.

o Let cool down the bread.

29. Simple keto breakfast with fried eggs

Total Time: 10 mins | Serving 1

Calories: Kcal 425, Fat:41g, Net Carbs:1g Protein:13g

Ingredients

o Eggs 2

o Butter 1 tbsp

o Mayonnaise 2 tbsp

o Baby spinach 1 oz

o Ground black pepper & salt

o Coffee or tea 1 cup

Steps of Preparation

o   Heat butter over med heat in a frying pan.

o   Crack the eggs into the pan right away. For sunny side up eggs, -leaving one side of the eggs to fry. Cooked over quick for eggs-flip over the eggs after a couple of mins and cook for 1 more minute. Only stop the cooking for a few more mins for stronger yolks. Season with pepper and salt

o   Serve a dollop of mayonnaise with baby spinach.

2.30. Keto taco omelet

Total Time: 20 mins |Serving 2

Calories: Kcal 797, Fat:63g, Net Carbs:8g Protein:44g

Ingredients

Taco seasoning

o   Onion powder ¼ tsp

o   Ground cumin ½ tsp

o   Paprika powder ½ tsp

o   Garlic powder ½ tsp

o   Chili flakes ¼ tsp

o   Salt ½ tsp

o   Ground black pepper ¼ tsp

o   Fresh oregano ½ tsp

Omelet

o   Ground beef 5 oz

o   Large eggs 4

o   Olive oil 1 tbsp

o   Avocado 1

o   Shredded cheddar cheese 5 oz

o   Diced tomato 1

o   Fresh cilantro 1 tsp

o Sea salt ½ tsp

o Ground black pepper ¼ tsp

Steps of Preparation

o Combine all Taco Seasoning products.

o In a large non-stick pan, add the ground beef. Apply the seasoning mixture(taco), blend well, and fry till completely cooked. Set aside in the bowl and remove it from heat.

o Beat the eggs in a mixing bowl and brush until they are soft.

o Reduce heat and add the olive oil in the saucepan. And add the eggs. Push the edges into the center, enabling the uncooked pieces to spill to the side, while the edges become solid. Cook a couple of mins, keep the inside a little runny.

o At ground beef, pinch lime.

o Break avocado half. The pit is Removed and suck the flesh out. Split into fragments.

o Spread ground beef over the omelet. Apply 2/3 of the grilled diced cheese and tomatoes.

o Remove the omelet cautiously from the pan. Add more avocado, cheese, and cilantro. Season salt & pepper. Serve.

30. Keto dosa

Total Time: 25 mins | Serving 2

Calories: Kcal 356, Fat:33g, Net Carbs:4g Protein:12g

Ingredients

o Almond flour ½ cup

o Shredded mozzarella cheese 1½ oz

o Coconut milk ½ cup

o Ground cumin ½ tsp

o Ground coriander seed ½ tsp

o Salt

Steps of Preparation

o Mix All ingredients in a bowl.

- o Heat a non-stick skillet and oil lightly. The use of a non-stick skillet is very important to avoid the dosa from adhering to the pan.
- o Pour in and spread the batter, by the pan moving.
- o Cook on low heat the dosa. The cheese starts melting and crisping away.
- o Once all the way through, it is cooked, and the dosa has turned golden brown on a side using the spatula fold it.
- o Serve with chutney made from coconut.

For the Peanut Sauce:

- o Peanut butter 1/2 cup
- o Minced fresh ginger 1 tsp
- o Minced fresh garlic 1 tsp
- o Minced jalapeño pepper 1 Tbsp
- o Sugar-free fish sauce 1 tbsp
- o Sugar rice wine vinegar 2 tbsp
- o Lime juice 1 tbsp
- o Water 2 tbsp
- o Erythritol granulated (sweetener) 2 tbsp

Steps of Preparation

For the Chicken:

- o In a big bowl, Mix the fresh lemon juice, fish sauce, soy sauce, Rice vinegar, avocado oil, cayenne pepper, ginger, garlic, ground coriander & sweetener, and whisk.
- o Apply pieces of chicken and stir to thoroughly coat the chicken only with marinade.
- o Cover & chill up to twenty-four hrs., or for at least 1 hr.
- o Remove 1/2 hr. before cooking from the freezer & heat the grill.
- o Grill the chicken on med heat for around 6 to 8 mins each side.
- o Remove it from the grill, add peanut sauce & serve.
- o Chopped up cabbage, diced peanuts, minced scallions & minced cilantro are optional garnishes.

For the Sauce with Peanut:

o Mix all the ingredients from the sauce in a mixer & mix till smooth.

o Before serving, taste and set sweetness& saltiness to your choice.

31. One-Skillet Chicken with Lemon Garlic Cream Sauce
Total Time: 30 mins |Serving 4|

Ingredients

o Skinless &boneless chicken thighs 4

o Salt & pepper

o Chicken broth 1 cup

o Lemon juice 2 tbsp

o Minced garlic 1 tbsp

o Red pepper flakes ½ tsp

o Olive oil 1 tbsp

o Finely diced shallots ⅓ cup

o Salted butter 2 tbsp

o Heavy cream ¼ cup

o Chopped parsley 2 tbsp

Steps of Preparation

o The thighs or chicken breasts are pounded into 1/2-inch thickness using a mallet. Sprinkle both sides of the chicken with a pinch of salt & pepper.

o Mix the chicken broth, juice of lemon, red pepper flakes, & garlic into a two-cup measuring cup.

o Place a rack in the bottom 3rd of your oven & preheat to 375of.

o Heat the olive oil on med-high heat in the big oven-safe pan. Apply the chicken & let it to brown for 2 to 3 mins each side. Unless the chicken isn't fully cooked, don't worry, finish it in your oven. Take the chicken off to a plate.

o Decrease the flame-med, apply the shallots & the chicken broth combination to the pan. Drag the bottom of the skillet with a whisk, so that all brown pieces are loosened. Kick up the heat back to med height and let the sauce come to low heat. Continue cooking the sauce for 10 to 15 mins, or till the sauce stays about 1/3 cup.

o Take from the flame whenever the sauce has thickened, then apply the butter & whisk till it fully melts. Apply the heavy whipping cream with the pan off flame, whisk in to mix. Place the pan on the flame for only thirty sec, Do NOT let the sauce boil. Take away from heat, apply the chicken back into the skillet & sprinkle the chicken over the sauce. Put the pan 5 to 8 mins in the oven, or till the chicken is fully cooked. Season with minced parsley or basil & serve hot with extra slices of lemon.

32. Low Carb Chicken Enchilada (Green) Cauliflower Casserole

Total Time: 45 mins | Serving 1

Calories: Cal 311, Fat:18g, Net Carbs:4g Protein:33g

Ingredients

o Frozen cauliflower florets 20 oz

o Softened cream cheese 4 oz

o Shredded cooked chicken 2 cups

o Salsa Verde ½ cups

o Kosher salt 1/2 tsp

o Ground black pepper 1/8 tsp

o Cheddar cheese shredded 1 cup

o Sour cream 1/4 cup

Steps of Preparation

o Place the cauliflower in a safe microwave plate and bake for 10 to 12 mins or till the pork is soft.

o Before microwave for the next thirty sec, add the cream cheese.

o Stir in the chicken, green salsa, pepper, salt, sour cream, cilantro& cheddar cheese.

o Bake for twenty mins inside an ovenproof baking dish in a preheated oven at 190 °, or you could have a 10-minute microwave on high. Serve warm.

33. Chicken crust pizza guilt-free

Total Time: 40 mins | Serving 8

Ingredients

- **For Crust**
- Fresh chicken breast 1.5 lbs.
- Minced garlic 2-3 cloves
- Blend Italian spice 1.5 tsp
- Shredded parmesan cheese 1/3 cup
- Shredded mozzarella cheese 1/3 cup
- Large egg 1
- **For toppings**
- Pasta sauce 3-4 tbsp
- Veggies
- Shredded mozzarella cheese 1/2 cup
- Shredded parmesan cheese 1/2 cup

Steps of Preparation

- Oven preheated to 400 ° c.
- Split the raw chicken into one "cubes & place it in small batches in a food processor to create some kind of handmade ground chicken.
- Place the raw ground chicken & the garlic, Italian spices, cheeses & egg in a bowl. Mix well.
- Line a baking sheet with a bakery release paper. Place the raw chicken combination ball on paper.
- Move out that much plastic wrap to covering the full pan or sheet and put it on top of the chicken combination ball. Push the chicken combination until it fills the pan or sheet.
- Pushed into two baking sheets for a lighter, crispier crust.
- Bake for almost 15 to 25 mins at 400 °, or till the crust becomes golden & to the desired crispness. Thicker crusts would be more about 20 to 25 mins & thin crusts take to cook in 10 to 15 mins.
- Take from the oven allow it to cool for around five mins.
- Distribute the sauce & top with the mozzarella. Apply the toppings & finish with the parmesan.
- Cook for 10 to 15 mins at 400 °, or till cheese seasoning has browned slightly.
- Cut, serve & enjoy this high protein meal that's free of guilt, low carb!

34. Asparagus stuffed chicken with parmesan

Servings: 3 | Total time: 30 min

Calories: 230 kcal | Proteins: 62 g | Carbohydrates: 10 g | Fat: 31 g

Ingredients

o   Chicken Breasts 3

o   Garlic paste 1 teaspoon

o   Asparagus 12 Stalks

o   Cream Cheese 1/2 cup

o   Butter 1 tablespoon

o   Olive Oil 1 teaspoon

o   Marinara Sauce 3/4 cup

o   shredded Mozzarella 1 cup

o   Salt and Pepper

Steps of Preparation

o   To start cooking the chicken, swirl the chicken (or split it in half without slicing it all

the way around. The chicken breast can open like a butterfly with one end already intact in the center). Remove the asparagus stalks and set it aside.

o   Rub salt, some pepper, and garlic all across the chicken breasts (both in and out). Divide the cream cheese between all the chicken breasts and then spread to the inside. Now place four stalks of asparagus and afterward fold one side of that same breast over another, wrapping it in place with the help of a toothpick to ensure that it doesn't get open.

o   Now preheat the oven, then set it to a broiler. Then Add butter and the olive oil to a hot saucepan and put the chicken breasts in it. Now took the breasts on either side for almost 6-7 minutes (the overall period would be 14-15 minutes based on the size of the breast) until the chicken will be almost cooked through.

o   Now top each breast with almost 1/4 cup of marinara sauce and also top with shredded mozzarella. Put in the oven and bake

Chapter 3: Keto lunch recipes for women over 50

For women over 50 trying the keto diet, these simple keto lunch recipes are great and will help to get a balanced fat ketosis.

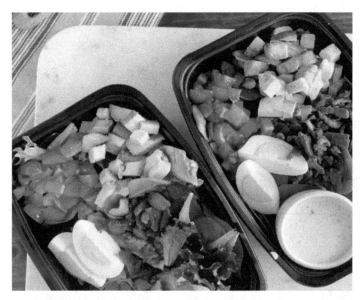

1. Keto avocado salad served with Blackened shrimp

Servings: 2 yields | Total time: 20 min

Calories: 420 kcal | Proteins: 49.5 g | Carbohydrates: 21 g | Fat: 18.5 g

Ingredients

- One teaspoon crushed basil
- One teaspoon black pepper
- One teaspoon cayenne
- Half kilogram peeled large shrimp
- Two minced cloves of garlic
- Two teaspoons paprika
- One teaspoon dehydrated thyme
- One teaspoon salt
- Two bunches of Asparagus
- One teaspoon of olive oil

- o Four cups lettuce leaves
- o One Avocado, diced
- o One fourth red onion, cut
- o One handful of basil leaves
- o One third cup greek yogurt
- o One teaspoon lemon pepper
- o One teaspoon lemon extract
- o Two tablespoons of water
- o Salt as required

Steps of preparation

- o In a narrow container, transfer shrimp and all other ingredients, and evenly coated it. Heat a big on medium flame and add some olive oil. Sauté the shrimp or prawns and the Asparagus, keep on turning seldom until they change color.
- o Now combine the lettuce leaves, the avocado, the onion slices, and the basil leaves in a glass bowl. Now add the shrimp or prawns and avocado. Add some dressing.
- o For the preparation of dressing, mix yogurt with the lemon pepper, the lemon juice, and the water and salt. Mix them well.

2. Keto Easy Egg Wrap lunch

Servings: 2 yields | Total time: 5 min

Calories: 411 kcal | Proteins: 25 g | Carbohydrates: 3 g | Fat: 31 g

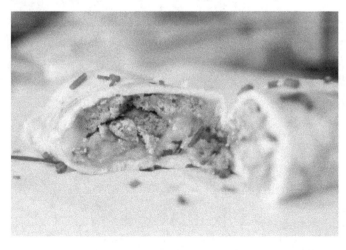

Ingredients

- o Two Eggs
- o Boiled turkey
- o Mashed Avocado,
- o Crushed Cheese
- o Half teaspoon pepper,
- o Half teaspoon paprika,
- o Hummus
- o A pinch of salt
- o A pinch of cayenne pepper

Steps of preparation

- o Heat a shallow skillet over a medium heat. Use   Butter or oil to grease.
- o Break one egg in a dish and blend well and with a fork.
- o Drop it in a hot skillet and tilt it to spread the egg into a wide circle at the bottom of the pan.
- o Let it simmer for 30 seconds.
- o Switch sides gently with a huge spatula and let it cook for the next 30 seconds.
- o Remove from heat and replicate the process for as number of eggs as you like to make.
- o Let the egg wraps cool down slightly (or completely), cover with the fillings as needed, wrap and serve it hot or cold.

3. Keto California Turkey and Bacon Lettuce Wraps with Basil-Mayo

Servings: 4 | Total time: 45 min

Calories: 303 kcal | Proteins: 11 g | Carbohydrates: 25 g | Fat: 20 g

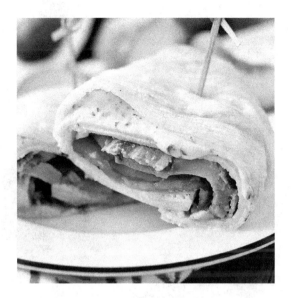

Ingredients

o One iceberg lettuce

o Four slices of deli turkey

o Four slices bacon

o One diced avocado

o One thinly diced tomato

o Half cup mayonnaise

o Six basil leaves

o One teaspoon lemon extract

o One chopped garlic clove

o Salt as desired

o Pepper as desired

Steps of preparation

o To prepare Basil-Mayo, mix the ingredients in a food processor and process till smooth. n Optionally, mince both the basil and the garlic and mix them all together. This can be done in a couple of days ahead.

o Place two wide leaves of lettuce on One slice of turkey and drench with Basil-Mayo. Put on a thin slice of turkey accompanied by bacon, including a couple of slices of avocado and the tomato. Season gently with salt and pepper, and then curl the bottom up as well as the sides in and roll it like a burrito. Cut halfway through, and then serve it cold.

4. Keto Lasagna Stuffed Portobellos

Servings: 4 yields | Total time: 25 min

Calories: 482 kcal | Proteins: 28 g | Carbohydrates: 6.5 g | Fat: 36 g

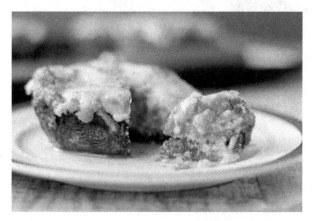

Ingredients

o   Four mushrooms

o   Four Italian sausage

o   One milk mozzarella cheese

o   One chopped parsley

o   One cup of whole milk cheese

o   One cup marinara sauce

Steps of preparation

o   Clean the mushrooms. Remove the branches using a spoon.

o   Take the sausage out and push the mixture into 4 patties. Force each patty into each of the mushroom cups, towards the edges and also up the sides of the Pattie.

o   Now put 1/4 cup of the ricotta in each of the mushroom caps and then press the sides of it, creating a hole in the middle.

o   Spoon 1/4 cup of sauce of marinara onto each mushroom on the highest point of the ricotta base.

o   Sprinkle 1/4 cup of sliced mozzarella cheese on the top.

o   Bake in a 375-degree F preheated oven for almost 40 minutes.

o   Garnish it with parsley and serve when warm.

5. Rapid Keto Sushi

Servings: 3 yields | Total time: 25 min

Calories: 353 kcal | Proteins: 18.3 g | Carbohydrates: 5.7 g | Fat: 5.7 g

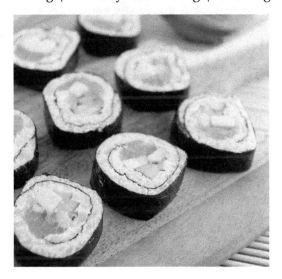

Ingredients

o   One nori wrapper

o   One cup of sliced cauliflower

o   Half avocado

o   One and a half oz Cream Cheese

o   One fourth cup cucumber

o   One tablespoon coconut oil

o   One cup of soy sauce

Steps of preparation

o   Split about half the head of the cauliflower into the florets and spin in the processor until the rice is appropriately smooth.

o   Heat the coconut oil in a medium-high pan and introduce the cauliflower rice.

o   Then Cook for almost 5-7 minutes till the rice is finely golden brown and cooked completely. Put it in a separate bowl.

o Slice the avocado, the cream cheese, and the cucumber into thinly sliced pieces and put them aside with the prepared cauliflower rice.

o Place a long sheet of plastic wrap on a clear, flat surface and place the nori wrapping above the plastic wrap.

o Cover the cauliflower rice over all the nori wrapping as thinly or as dense as you want in an even coating. Leave some room around the corners and edges.

o For some keto sushi rice, apply the first coating of the avocado on the rice adjacent to you. Next, add a thin layer of some cream cheese straight to the avocado, and finally, add a layer of cucumber.

o For keto sushi cucumber, firs raise the plastic wrap on the side by using your palms to mask the ingredients.

o Steadily stretch the plastic wrap and the nori wraps over the avocado, the cucumber, and the cream cheese before you cover the whole.

o Using a sharp knife, split the sushi into eight parts. First, Begin in the center so that the rice is not pulled out along with the weight of the knife.

6. Chicken Piccata keto Meatballs

Serving: 3 | Total: Time 30 min

Calories: 323 kcal, Fat:21g, Net Carbs:2g Protein:26g

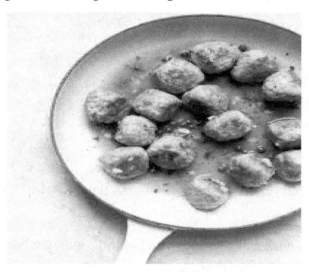

Ingredients

- o Ground chicken 1 lb.
- o Almond flour 1/3 cup
- o Egg 1
- o Kosher salt 1/2 tsp
- o Ground black pepper 1/4 tsp
- o Garlic powder 1/4 tsp
- o Lemon zest 1/2 tsp
- o Fresh chopped parsley 1 tsp
- o Olive oil 2 tbsp

For the sauce:

- o Dry white wine 1/2 cup
- o Lemon juice 2 tbsp
- o Drained & chopped capers 2 tbsp
- o Lemon zest 1/4 tsp
- o Butter 1/4 cup

Steps of Preparation

- o In a med bowl, mix the ground meat, almond meal/flour, egg, pepper, salt, powder of garlic, zest of the lemon as well as parsley together & stir thoroughly. Form into fifteen meatballs. Heat the oil of olive in a non-stick skillet & cook the meatballs till they become golden brown & fried through.
- o In the same skillet as the meatballs were cooked, add the white wine & bring to a simmer, having to scrape all the meatballs off the skillet & into the white wine. Apply the juice of lemon & capers and reduce by around half (2 to 3 mins). Turn off the heat & stir in the zest of lemon & butter till melted as well as smooth. sprinkle with salt to taste

7. Keto Chicken Alfredo Spaghetti Squash

Servings: 4 | Total Time: 20 mins

Calories: 327 kcal | Fat:25g | Net Carbs:14g | Protein:12g

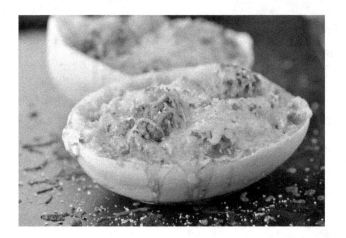

Ingredients

o   2 tbsp butter

o   Minced Garlic 2 tsp

o   Sage 1 tsp

o   Flour 2tbsp

o   Chicken broth 1 cup

o   Half cream 1/2 cup

o   Cubed cream cheese 4 oz

o   Shredded parmesan cheese ½ cup

o   Cooked & shredded chicken 1/2 cup

o   Cooked spaghetti squash 2 1/2 cups

o   Pepper, salt & parsley

Steps of Preparation

o   Melt the butter over med-heat in a pan.

o   Add the sage & garlic, then cook for around a min.

o   Mix in the flour/meal & cook, constantly mixing for around a minute.

o   Mix a half & half in a chicken broth.

o   Mix in the parmesan cheese & cream cheese till smooth.

o   Add the vegetable squash, cooked and shredded chicken, & cook till fully heated.

o   Taste the alfredo vegetable squash with chicken, then top with pepper, salt & parsley.

8. Keto Paleo lunch Spice Chicken Skewers

Serving 2 | Total Time: 2 hours

Calories: 198 | Fat:5g | Net Carbs |1g Protein:35g

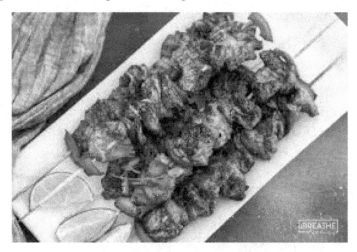

Ingredients

o   Boneless & skinless chicken tenders 2 lb.

o   Granulated erythritol sweetener 2 tbsp

o   5 spice powder 2 tbsp

o   Rice wine vinegar unsweetened 1 tbsp

o   Avocado oil 1 tbsp

o   Sesame oil 1 tsp

o   Gluten-free soy sauce 1 tbsp

o   Skewers red bell pepper pieces 1 cup

o   Skewers 12

Steps of Preparation

o   Cut the chicken finely into pieces just around two inches long onto the diagonal.

o   In a med bowl, mix the sweetener, five powder spice, rice wine vinegar, oil of avocado, oil of sesame, soy sauce & cayenne pepper & stir.

o   Season & adjust sweetness/saltiness according to your preference.

o   Apply the pieces of chicken, then mix well to coat.

o   Marinate a chicken for one hr. or more, & up to twenty-four hrs.

- Heat the grill.

- Thread pieces of chicken & red bell pepper onto the skewers.

- Grill each side for 2 -3 mins or once the chicken is cooked through.

- When desired, garnish with lime slices & cilantro (fresh).

9. Keto Asian pork ribs

| Serving 4 | Total Time 1 hr.

Calories: 505 | Fat: 44g | Net Carbs: 1g | Protein: 25g

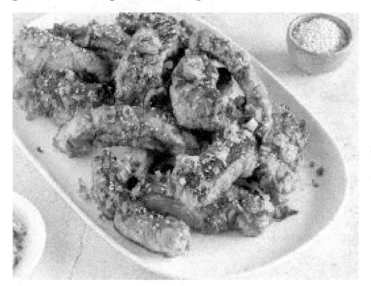

Ingredients

- Chopped pork spareribs into individual ribs 2 lb.

- Fresh diced ginger 1 tbsp

- Diced green onions 2 tbsp

- Szechuan peppercorns ½ tbsp

- 2-star anise

- Diced garlic cloves 3

- Gluten-free tamari sauce or coconut amino 2 tbsp

- Avocado oil 2 tbsp

- Salt & pepper to taste

Steps of Preparation

- To a big pot of boiling water, add flour, Szechuan peppercorns, star anise, & ribs. Bring to boil, then cook till the meat is soft, for 45 mins. Skim away any shaping foam.

- Drain from the pot & remove ribs. Remove the star anise & peppercorns.

- Apply the avocado oil to the frying pan, then add the ginger and garlic. Put in ribs & cook on the medium-high fire. Add the coconut amino or tamari sauce, then season, to taste, with pepper and salt.

- Stir-fry ribs over high heat until fully covered and browned with the sauce.

10. Keto slow cooker pork's rib (Asian)

Servings: 2 | Total Time:3hrs. 20 mins

Calories: 482 | Fat: 38g | Net Carbs: 4g | Protein: 25g

Ingredients

- Baby back pork ribs 450g
- Sliced medium onion 1/2
- Garlic paste 1 tbsp
- Ginger paste 1 tbsp
- Chicken broth 1&1/2 c
- Gluten-free tamari sauce or coconut amino 2 tbsp
- Chinese five-spice seasoning ½ tsp
- Sliced green onions 2

Steps of Preparation

- Place the pork ribs rack inside the slow cooker. The rack may need to be halved to fit.

- Include the onions, paste for garlic, paste for the ginger, and broth for the meat. If the ribs are not completely coated, add up a little bit of broth until covered.

- Cover & cook for three hours at low flame.

- To keep warm, remove ribs & wrap in foil. Place this apart.

- Shift the onions & products from the slow cooker into the stove to a clean pan. Using a hand blender, blitz well (or use a food processor to blitz and move to the stove in the pan) and apply the Chinese 5-spice & tamari. Reduce the paste to dense and jammy, over a relatively high flame.

- o Taste the marinade and add in a bit of erythritol if you think it will improve from a little more sugar.
- o Brush over the warm ribs with this marinade & garnish with onions.

11. Keto baked ribs recipe

Serving 2 | Total Time: 3hrs. 5 mins

Calories 580 | Fat: 51g | Net Carbs: 5g | Protein: 25g

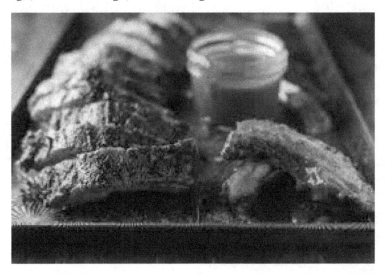

Ingredients

- o Baby back ribs 1 lb.
- o Applesauce 2 tbsp
- o Gluten-free tamari sauce or coconut amino 2 tbsp
- o Olive oil 2 tbsp
- o Fresh ginger 1 tbsp
- o Garlic cloves 2
- o Salt & pepper

Steps of Preparation

- o Preheat the oven to 275 F– change it to the minimum temperature if your oven does not go down to this point.
- o Season with salt & pepper over ribs & cover securely with foil. Put the product onto a baking dish and bake in the oven for three hours at low temp.

- Mix olive oil, applesauce, tamari sauce, ginger, and garlic in a blender until it creates a purée.

- Take the ribs out from the oven after three hours, then adjust the heat in the oven up to 450 F (230 C) or just as high as the oven can go.

- With care, open the foil so the ribs can rest on top of the foil. Coat the ribs well with the marinade, by using a brush. Put the ribs in the oven and bake for 5-10 mins till it becomes sticky with marinade.

12. Keto fried pork tenderloin

Serving 2 | Total Time: 20 mins

Calories: 389 Kcal | Fat: 23g | Net Carbs: 0g | Protein: 47g

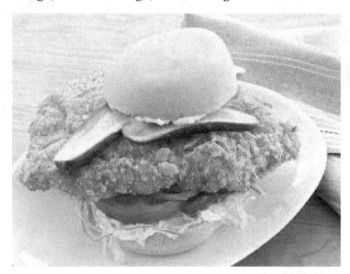

Ingredients

- Pork tenderloin 1 lb.
- Salt & pepper>> to taste
- Avocado or coconut oil 2 tbsp

Steps of Preparation

- Break the pork tenderloin into two-three pieces to fit more conveniently into your frying pan.

- Apply the oil to the frying pan & fry the pork tenderloin first on one side, using tongs. Using tongs, flip the pork tenderloin until that side is fried, then cook the other side until both sides are browned.

o Continue to turn the pork every several minutes till the meat thermometer displays just below 145F (63C), internal temperature. Since you remove it from the frying pan, the pork will begin to cook a little.

o Let the pork rest for a couple of minutes then slice with a knife into one-inch-thick slices.

13. Cauliflower Grits with shrimps and Arugula

Servings: 4 yields | Total time: 30 min

Calories: 122 kcal | Proteins: 16 g | Carbohydrates: 3 g | Fat: 5 g

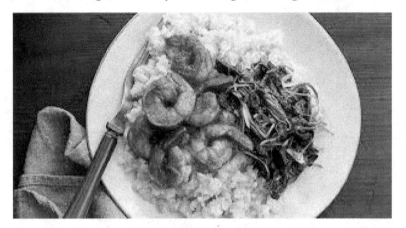

Ingredients

o One-pound peeled shrimp

o One tablespoon bell pepper crushed

o Two teaspoons garlic paste

o Half teaspoon cayenne pepper

o One tablespoon olive oil

o Salt and freshly ground black pepper

o One tablespoon butter

o Four cups riced cauliflower

o One cup milk

o Half cup crumbled goat cheese

o Salt and freshly ground black pepper

o One tablespoon olive oil

o Three diced garlic cloves

- Four cups arugula
- Salt and black pepper as desired

Steps of preparation

- Put the shrimp in a big plastic zip bag. In a medium container, mix the paprika with some garlic powder and the cayenne. Put the mixture to the shrimp bag and toss well until the spices are covered. Refrigerate when you're preparing the grits.
- Melt the butter in a medium pot over medium heat. Include the cauliflower rice and cook till some moisture is produced, that is 2 to 3 minutes.
- Mix in half milk and bring to boil. Allow it to boil, keep stirring regularly, until some milk is absorbed by the cauliflower for; it will happen in 6 to 8 minutes.
- Incorporate the leftover milk and boil until the mixture is dense and smooth, cook for 10 minutes. Mix with goat cheese and then season it with some salt and pepper. Keep it warm.

14. Keto Chipotle Pork Wraps

Servings: 2 yields | Total time: 15 min

Calories: 292 kcal | Proteins: 14 g | Carbohydrates: 37 g | Fat: 0 g

Ingredients

- Half Avocado
- Two tablespoons Mayonnaise
- One lime juice extract
- One clove of garlic minced
- Salt and pepper as required
- Water
- One Head Iceberg Lettuce
- Two cups Pork
- One Avocado

Steps of preparation

- Mash the avocado and sweep in the mayonnaise, garlic, lime juice, and some salt and pepper. If the aioli wants to be thin, then apply a little bit of water so that it can be quickly drizzled.

o Place the pork in the lettuce cups, cover with the sliced avocado, and drizzle it with the aioli and cover with cilantro and some lime.

15. Keto Italian Chicken Meal Prep Bowls

Servings: 2 yields | Total time: 15 min

Calories: 292 kcal | Proteins: 14 g | Carbohydrates: 37 g | Fat: 0 g

Ingredients

o One teaspoon salt
o half t teaspoon pepper
o Two teaspoon basil
o Two teaspoon marjoram
o Two teaspoon rosemary
o Two teaspoon thyme
o Two teaspoons paprika
o Two pounds boneless skinless chicken breasts cut into bite-sized pieces
o One and a half cup broccoli florets
o One small red chopped onion
o One cup tomato
o One medium zucchini chopped
o Two teaspoons minced garlic
o Two Tablespoon olive oil
o Two cups cooked rice

Steps of preparation

o Preheat the oven to 450F. Then Line the baking sheet of aluminum foil and put it aside.
o In a small container, add some salt, some pepper, marjoram, some rosemary, basil, thyme, and paprika.
o Put chicken and vegetables in the baking bowl. Spray all the seasoning and garlic equally over all the chicken as well as the vegetables. Then Drizzle with some olive oil.
o Now Bake for almost 15-20 minutes unless the chicken is properly cooked and vegetables are finely crispy.

- o Broil the brown chicken for 1-2 minutes.
- o Put 1/2 or 1 cup of the cooked rice of your preference in four different preparation containers.
- o Segregate chicken and vegetables equally all over the rice.
- o Cover them, and them keep in the refrigerator for 3-5 days, or you can serve them for dinner.

16. Cheeseburger Lettuce Wraps

Servings: 1 | Total time: 15 min

Calories: 556 kcal | Proteins: 33.6 g | Carbohydrates: 8.2 g | Fat: 42 g

Ingredients

- o Two pounds minced beef
- o Half teaspoon salts
- o One teaspoon black pepper
- o One teaspoon oregano
- o Six slices of American cheese
- o Two heads iceberg
- o Two tomatoes diced
- o One fourth cup light mayo
- o Three tablespoons ketchup
- o One Tablespoon relish
- o salt and pepper as required

Steps of preparation

- o First, heat the grill or the skillet over medium temperature.
- o In a large container, add some ground beef, some seasoned salt, and pepper, and some oregano.
- o Now Divide the mixture into six parts and then curl each of them into a ball. Squeeze each ball down to create a patty.
- o Put the patties on the grill or the pan and then cook for almost 4 minutes from either direction or till cooked to desired taste. (when using a grill, just prepare 3 min at a time to avoid congestion).

o Put a piece of cheese on top of the grilled burgers. Put each cheeseburger on a broad lettuce leaf. Cover with spreading and one slice of tomato, some red onion, and whatever you want. Wrap the lettuce over the top then eat. Savor it!

o In a little pan, add all the components of the spread. Put it in the fridge before available for usage.

17. Classic Stuffed Peppers

Servings: 6 | Total time: 1 hour 20 min

Calories: 376 kcal | Proteins: 16 g | Carbohydrates: 52 g | Fat: 12 g

Ingredients

o Six bell peppers

o One-pound ground beef

o One minced onion

o Two minced garlic cloves

o Three fourth cup boiled rice

o One teaspoon paprika

o Half teaspoon oregano

o Half teaspoon mustard powder

o Half cup parsley

o Salt and black pepper

o Half cup Jack cheese

Steps of preparation

o Preheat to 375 ° F in the oven. Apply the marinara sauce to the center of a medium-sized skillet.

o Prune the base within each pepper a bit, so it lies flat. Break off the tops of each pepper and then detach the ribs and the seeds and then discard them.

o In a medium dish, combine beef with onion, paprika, oregano, garlic, rice, mustard pepper, and some parsley and salt

o Load the mixture of meat into each of the peppers, filling up to the top. Shift the peppers to the heated skillet and put them on the upper edge of the sauce.

o   Garnish with one and a half teaspoons of cheese. Bake until the peppers are juicy, and the beef is thoroughly cooked for 25 to 30 minutes. Serve straight away with some scoop of sauce.

18. Chicken Lemon herb Mediterranean salad

Servings: 1 | Total time: 15 min

Calories: 336 kcal | Proteins: 24 g | Carbohydrates: 13 g | Fat: 21 g

Ingredients

o   Two tablespoons olive oil

o   One lemon juice extract

o   Two tablespoons of water

o   Two tablespoons of vinegar

o   Two tablespoons of parsley

o   Two teaspoons basil

o   Two teaspoons of minced garlic

o   Two teaspoons of oregano

o   One teaspoon of salt

o   One pepper

o   One-pound boneless chicken thigh fillets

o   Four cups Romaine lettuce leaves

o   One diced cucumber

o   Two tomatoes cubed

o   One red onion cubed

o   One diced avocado

o   One-third cup rutted Kalamata olives

Steps of preparation

o   In a big container, mix together all the marinade components. Add half of the marinade to a big, shallow pan. Refrigerate the leftover marinade for further use as a topping.

o In a bowl, add chicken to some marinade and marinate the chicken for 15-30 minutes (and for up to 2 hours in the fridge if time allows). When waiting for the chicken to marinate, arrange all the components of the salad, and combine in a big bowl of salad.

o When chicken is prepared, warm 1 tablespoon of olive oil inside a grill pan or grill above medium-high heat. Barbecue chicken from both sides until golden brown and cooked completely.

o Keep chicken to settle for 5 min; cut and place over the salad. Drizzle with the leftover unchanged dressing. End up serving with a lemon slice.

19. Keto BLT stuffed chicken salad avocados

Servings: 1 | Total time: 30 min

Calories: 267 kcal | Proteins: 14 g | Carbohydrates: 13.6 g | Fat: 17 g

Ingredients

o Twelve slices of turkey bacon

o One and a half cups of shredded rotisserie chicken

o Two tomatoes

o One and a half cups of cottage cheese

o One cup of finely chopped lettuce

o Three avocados

Steps of preparation

o Preheat the oven to the temperature of 400 degrees F.

o Place Twelve slices of the turkey bacon on a parchment lining the baking dish

o Bake for almost 10 minutes, then rotate, and bake for the next five minutes, then scatter the bacon over a few sheets of some paper towels to it cool off.

o In the meantime, quarter the tomatoes, scrape out all the pulp and the seeds with the help of fingertips, and break into tiny bits.

o Cut the Romaine into little bits

o In a big bowl, add meat, some cottage cheese, some romaine, some berries, turkey bacon, and combine together.

o Sprinkle with salt and pepper as desired.

- Half the avocados cut the pits and then season gently with some salt and pepper.
- Scoop 1/6 (roughly) of the chicken salad inside each avocado. Not a massive amount is going to fit into the hole produced by the seed, so you're going to add a good amount on upper edge of the avocado.

20. Cheesy taco skillet

Servings: 6 yields | Total time: 30 min

Calories: 241 kcal | Proteins: 30 g | Carbohydrates: 9 g | Fat: 20 g

Ingredients

- One-pound ground beef
- One diced large yellow onion
- Two diced bell peppers
- One diced tomato
- One shredded large zucchini
- taco seasoning
- Three cups pf baby kale
- One and a half cup of shredded cheddar cheese

Steps of preparation

- In a wide pan, gently cook ground beef and also well crumble.
- Drain the waste of fat.
- Include the onions and the peppers and cook till golden.
- Add some canned tomatoes, some taco seasoning, as well as any water required for taco seasoning to uniformly cover the mixture (up to 1 tablespoon – the tomato liquid may benefit)
- Apply the greens and make it absolutely wilt.
- Mix it finely.

21. Cauliflower Cheesy Breadsticks

Servings: 8 | Total time: 43 min

Calories: 102 kcal | Proteins: 7.1 g | Carbohydrates: 1.1 g | Fat: 7.7 g

Ingredients

o Four cups of diced cauliflower

o Four eggs

o Two cups of mozzarella

o Three teaspoon oregano

o Four minced cloves of garlic

o Salt and pepper as desired

o One cup of mozzarella cheese

Steps of preparation

o Start by Preheating the oven to a temperature of 425 ° F. Arrange Two pizza plates or a broad baking sheet with parchment paper on them.

o Try to make sure the florets of cauliflower are finely cut. Apply the florets to the processor and spin.

o In a microwaveable jar, put the cauliflower then cover it with a lid. Microwave it for a time of 10-minutes. Only let cauliflower cool until there was no steam rising from it anymore. Put in a wide bowl the microwave cauliflower and transfer oregano, 2 cups mozzarella, salt, garlic, and pepper to the whites. Mix in everything.

o Segregate the mixture into two and put each half on the ready baking sheets and form the breadsticks either into a pizza crust or in a rectangular shape.

o Bake the crust for around 25 minutes (no covering yet) till it is soft and brown. Don't be scared; the crust isn't soggy. Sprinkle with the leftover mozzarella cheese once golden and bring it oven and bake for the next five min just until the cheese is melted.

o Start Slicing and serving.

22. Loaded cauliflower

Servings: 4 | Total time: 15 min

Calories: 298 kcal | Proteins: 7.4 g | Carbohydrates: 1.1 g | Fat: 24.6 g

Ingredients

o One-pound cauliflower

o Four ounces of sour cream

o   One cup of grated cheddar cheese

o   Two slices of bacon

o   Two tablespoons of chives

o   Three tablespoons of butter

o   One fourth teaspoon of garlic paste

o   Salt and pepper as required

Steps of preparation

o   Slice the cauliflower into the form of florets and transfer them to a suitable bowl within microwave. Add almost 2 teaspoons of water and soak with film that sticks. Microwave for another 5-8 minutes, before fully cooked and soft, based on the microwave. Dump the extra water and allow for a couple of seconds to stay uncovered. (Alternately, the traditional method, boil the cauliflower. Upon boiling, you can need to drain a little extra water out from inside the cauliflower.

o   In a food processor, add the cauliflower and process it until soft. Introduce the butter, and sour cream, and garlic powder, then process to the texture of mashed potatoes. Remove the mashed cauliflower to a pot and mix much of the chives, leaving any later to apply to the end. add the rest of the sharp cheddar cheese and combine through hand. Sprinkle some salt and pepper as desired.

o   Cover the filled cauliflower with the remainder cheese, leftover chives, and some bacon. To melt the cheese, place it in the microwave or place cauliflower for another few minutes under the broiler.

23. Keto Grilled tuna salad

Servings: 2 | Total time: 1 hour

Calories: 975 kcal | Proteins: 53 g | Carbohydrates: 9 g | Fat: 79 g

Ingredients

o   Two large egg

o   Eight ounces of asparagus

o   One tablespoon of olive oil

o   Eight ounces of fresh tuna

- o Four ounces of spring mix
- o Four ounces of cherry tomatoes
- o Half red onion
- o Two tablespoons of chopped walnuts
- o Half cup of mayonnaise
- o Two tablespoons of water
- o Two teaspoons of garlic paste
- o Salt and pepper were required

Steps for preparation

- o Gather all of the things for preparation.
- o Add the water, the garlic powder, mayonnaise, and salt, and the pepper together in a bowl to create the dressing. Mix until well blended and set it aside.
- o Boil the eggs for 8-10 minutes or so. Peel and break in half until cooled.
- o Clean and split the asparagus onto similar lengths. In a pan, cook the asparagus.
- o Pour the olive oil between both sides of the tuna in the same manner and fry it on both sides for 3-5 minutes. To taste, sprinkle the tuna with the salt and the pepper.
- o Put the leafy greens, the cherry tomatoes (sliced in half), onion, and the eggs on a tray.
- o Slice into pieces of the cooked tuna and put it on top. On the top of the salad, pour the dressing sauce and scatter the sliced walnuts on top of that.

24. Creamy ketogenic taco soup

Servings: 4 | Total time: 35 min

Calories: 345 kcal | Proteins: 21 g | Carbohydrates: 5 g | Fat: 27 g

Ingredients

- o Sixteen ounces of ground beef
- o One tablespoon of olive oil
- o One medium diced onion
- o Three minced cloves of garlic
- o One diced green bell pepper
- o Ten ounces of canned tomatoes

o   One cup of heavy cream

o   Two tablespoons of taco seasoning

o   Salt and pepper as required

o   Two cups of beef broth

o   One medium cubed avocado

o   Four tablespoons of sour cream

o   Four tablespoons of cilantro

Steps of preparation

o   Gather all of the supplies. Dice the bell pepper and the onion long in advance.

o   Add the olive oil, onion, and ground beef and garlic, to a small saucepan over medium heat. Sprinkle salt and pepper, season.

o   Cook it until golden brown beef and transparent onion.

o   Add some bell pepper, heavy cream, sliced tomatoes with green chili, and taco seasoning until the beef is golden brown.

o   Simmer together properly to guarantee that all of the products contain the spices and seasoning.

o   Transfer the water to the beef and then get the soup to a simmer. Decrease the heat to low and simmer for almost 10-15 minutes or until liquid is decreased, and soup is prepared according to the desired taste.   If needed, try and add salt and pepper.

o   Add the sour cream and the cilantro avocado to the portions and garnish. Add a   squeeze of lime juice, too.

25. Keto fish cakes with dipping sauce

Servings: 6 | Total time: 15 min

Calories: 69 kcal | Proteins: 53 g | Carbohydrates: 2.7 g | Fat: 6.5 g

Ingredients

o   One-pound raw white boneless fish

o   One by four cup of cilantro

o   Salt as required

o   Chili flakes as required

o   Two garlic cloves

o   Two tablespoons of coconut oil

o   Two ripe avocados

o   One lemon juice extract

o   Two tablespoons of water

Steps of preparation

o   Put the fish, vegetables, garlic (if used), spice, chili, and fish in a processor. Blitz before everything is equally mixed.

o   Apply the coconut oil to a wide frying pan over medium-high heat and stir the pan.

o   Oil the hands and roll in Six patties of the fish combination.

o   To the hot frying pan and add the cakes. Cook till lightly browned and fried thru, on both sides.

o   While the fish cakes are frying, in a blender, incorporate all the dipping sauce components (starting with lemon juice) and mix thoroughly until it becomes fluffy. Taste the mixture and apply, if necessary, other lemon juice or salt.

o   Serve hot with the dipping sauce when the fish cakes become baked.

26. Ketogenic Paleo Meat Ball for lunch

Servings: 3 | Total time: 30 min

Calories: 475 kcal | Proteins: 61.3 g | Carbohydrates: 5.6 g | Fat: 21.7 g

Ingredients

o   One and a half pounds of ground beef

o   Two tablespoons ghee

o   One tablespoon apple cider vinegar

o   Half teaspoon of pepper

o   One teaspoon of salt

o   Yellow minced onion

o   Two minced garlic cloved

o   One fourth cup of chopped rosemary

Steps of preparation

o   Start by Preheating the oven to the temperature of 350 degrees ° C.

- o Put all the meatballs supplies in a bowl and mix, and when well mixed, use the hands to combine it together.

- o Line a parchment paper on baking tray and fold the mixture into tiny balls, utilizing approximately a tablespoon of mix per meatball.

- o Now meatballs are wrapped and placed on the parchment. Bake for almost 20 minutes or until baked completely.

- o Serve hot or allow it to cool and seal in the refrigerator in an airtight jar.

27. Ketogenic Mexican Shredded beef

Servings: 20 | Total time: 3-hour 20 min

Calories: 323 kcal | Proteins: 53 g | Carbohydrates: 7.3 g | Fat: 12.9 g

Ingredients

- o Three and a half pounds beef short ribs
- o Two teaspoons turmeric powder
- o One teaspoon salt
- o Half teaspoon peppers
- o Two teaspoons cumin powder
- o Two teaspoons coriander powder
- o Half cup waters
- o One cup cilantro chopped

Steps of preparation

- o Combine the dried ingredients in a shallow pan.

- o For a slow cooker, introduce short ribs and gently brush each bit in the seasoning mix.

- o Scatter over the ribs with cilantro stems and additional garlic. Apply water carefully without scrubbing the spices off.

- o On low heat, cook for 6-7 hours, or until it falls apart. After 6 hours, inspect the beef and cook further when it's not soft enough.

- o Drain the cooking liquid in a medium pan if necessary and decrease it over a moderate flame for 15 minutes.

o Transfer the liquid back into another crockpot. Take off the steak and cut the beef utilizing two forks.

o Serve warm with guacamole, taco-like silverbeet leaves, corn, cucumbers, organic cilantro, and green beans.

28. Keto low carb pork & cashew stir fry

Total Time: 10 mins | Servings: 2 |

Calories: 403 kcal | Fat: 27g | Net Carbs: 12g | Protein: 28g

Ingredients

o Avocado oil 2 tbsp

o Shredded pork ½ lb.

o Sliced green bell pepper ½

o Sliced red bell pepper ½

o Sliced medium onion 1/4

o Cashews 1/3 c

o Fresh grated ginger 1 tbsp

o Minced cloves of garlic 3

o Chinese chili oil 1 tsp

o Sesame oil 1 tbsp

o Gluten-free tamari sauce or coconut amino 2 tbsp

o Salt>> to taste

Steps of Preparation

o Put avocado oil in a frying saucepan & cook the pork (if uncooked).

o Next, add onions, pepper & cashews, all sliced.

o Sauté until completely cooked pork. Then mix in ginger, garlic, tamari sauce, chili oil, sesame oil & salt to your taste.

29. Keto pork stuffed with sausages & cauliflower rice

Total Time: 30 mins | Serving 4
Calories: kcal 473 | Fat: 24g | Net Carbs: 3g | Protein: 57g

Ingredients

- o Avocado oil 4 tbsp
- o Minced garlic cloves 2
- o Small cauliflower cut into small rice-like particles ¼
- o Chopped onion 1 tbsp
- o Chopped red bell pepper 1 tbsp
- o Chopped sausage ½
- o Green peas 1 tbsp
- o Pork tenderloin 1&1/2 lb.
- o Salt & pepper>> to taste

Steps of Preparation

- o Preheat the oven before 400 F (200 C).
- o Pour 2 Tsp of avocado oil over moderate temp in a wide skillet, then add garlic & onion. Cook them, till the onion is transparent, for a few minutes.
- o Stir in the cauliflower, sausage, red pepper & roast for ten minutes. Season with salt & pepper.
- o Slice the pork tenderloin to open it lengthwise but don't cut through.   Using a meat pounder, pound meat if you've it.
- o Cover with rice mixture halfway over the tenderloin. Wrap meat up & use twine to bind it together. (use cocktail sticks to protect the pork If you don't have twine.)
- o In a separate frying pan, melt two tbsp of avocado oil. Crisp up the pork tenderloin gently on either side for a few minutes until it is brown.
- o Place your filled pork tenderloin upon the baking tray and let them steam for at least thirty minutes uncovered. If you have got a meat thermometer, this should display 145 F.
- o Let the meat sit for ten minutes before the strings are cut and sliced.

30. Keto pork tenderloin stuffed with cabbage

Total Time: 40 mins | Serving: 4

Calories: 207 kcal | Fat: 12g | Net Carbs: 2g | Protein: 24g

Ingredients

- o Avocado oil 2 tbsp
- o Diced onion ¼

o Diced cabbage 1 c

o Minced garlic cloves 2

o Salt & pepper>> to taste

o Pork tenderloin 1 lb.

Steps of Preparation

o Preheat the oven before 400 F (200 C).

o Apply the avocado oil over medium heat to a frying pan and sauté the cabbage, onions, garlic till cabbage is soft. Season to taste, with salt & black pepper.

o Lengthwise slit the tenderloin but do not cut into it all the way completely. Using it to hammer the pork tenderloin to a big flat slice (approx. 1/2-inch-thick), if you have got a meat pounder.

o Place the flat tenderloin over a cutting board & put the fried cabbage in the center.

o Roll up and cover the tenderloin with twine or use cocktail sticks to roast.

o Place it on a baking dish and take 40 mins. Testing the pork achieves an inner temp of 145 F.

31. Keto marinated pork tenderloin

Total Time: 20 mins | Serving 4

Calories: 258 kcal | Fat: 19g | Net Carbs: 1g | Protein: 24g

Ingredients

o Cut into 2 long pieces of pork tenderloin 1lb.

o Olive oil ¼ c

o Greek seasoning 2 tbsp

o Red wine vinegar 1 tbsp

o Lemon juice 1 tbsp

o Salt & pepper

for Greek Seasoning:

o Garlic powder 1 tsp

o Dried oregano 1tsp

o Dried basil 1tsp

o Dried rosemary ½ tsp

o Dried thyme ½ tsp

o Dried dill ½ tsp

o Cinnamon ½ tsp

o Parsley ½ tsp

o Marjoram ½ tsp

Steps of Preparation

o Mix the olive oil, vinegar, lemon juice & seasoning in a big zip lock container.

o Put the 2 pieces of pork tenderloin in the container and marinate in the fridge overnight.

o Place the pork over medium heat in a frying pan. Place the pork with one side and roast. Then by using tongs, turn the pork into a good browning on every side.

o Continue to turn the pork till the inner temp reaches 145 F/63 C (control using a meat thermometer).

32. Keto herbs pork tenderloin

Total Time: 20 mins | Serving 2

Total Time: kcal: 627 | Fat: 49g | Net Carbs: 4g | Protein: 44g

Ingredients

o Pine nut 2 tbsp

o Chopped garlic cloves 3

o Fresh basil leaves 1 c

o Fresh parsley ½ c + 2 tbsp

o Nutritional yeast 2 tbsp

o Olive oil 5 tbsp

o Juice of 1 lemon

o salt to taste

For the pork

o Pork tenderloin 14 oz

o Salt & ground black pepper

o Olive oil 1 tbsp

o   Reserved herbs paste 3 tbsp

Steps of Preparation

o   Begin by toasting pine nuts in a heavy, dry skillet to create the herb paste. Take out the crispy pine nuts and apply the garlic, basil, nutritional yeast flakes, fresh parsley, and olive oil to a mini food processor. Combine to make a perfect paste, scraping many times across the sides of the container. Season with salt & lemon juice to taste. Place on the side.

o   Preheat oven to 410 ° F (210 ° C) for pork.

o   Season the pork tenderloin on both sides with salt and freshly ground black pepper. In a non-stick pan, heat the olive oil & brown the tenderloin at both sides. Remove from heat and let it cool down a little bit. Using a palette knife or thin silicone spatula until cool enough to treat, then spread the stored herb paste over the pork tenderloin on both sides. Put tenderloin with a well-equipped cover in a casserole dish & cook in the oven for 12-15 mins or till cooked to your taste.

o   Remove from oven and enable it to cool before sliced and served. Serve with some extra herbs paste if needed.

33. Keto basil pork Fettucine

Total Time: 15 mins | Servings: 3

Calories: 231 | Fat: 16g | Net Carbs: 5g | Protein: 16g

Ingredients

o   5 packs of fettuccine shirataki noodles of 3 oz

o   coconut oil 2 tbsp

o   Pork tenderloin ½ lb.

o   salt & pepper>> to taste

o   Sliced leek 1

o   Chopped garlic cloves 2

o   coconut cream 4 tbsp

o   Fresh chopped basil leaves ¼ c

o   Dash of chicken broth

Steps of Preparation

o   To 400 F, preheat the oven.

o   Rinse under cool, flowing water the shirataki noodles, and hold warm in a pot of softly simmering water upon a burner.

o   Heat 1 tbsp of coconut oil in a wide saucepan and brown both sides of the pork tenderloin. Take the pork off the skillet & season with salt & black pepper. Shift the pork to a baking tray and put over it in the oven for ten min. Remove, and then let rest.

o   Meanwhile, heat in the same pan the remaining coconut oil used for the pork & cook the leeks & garlic over medium heat until soft. For keeping the mixture moist, apply a splash of chicken broth. Apply the coconut cream & basil once wet.

o   Drain the hot noodles and put them in a bowl. Spoon over sauce with leek. Cut the pork & put it on top of the sauce.

o

Chapter 4: Keto Dinner Recipes for Women above 50

These are some keto dinner recipes for women above 50. These recipes are simple, easy, and fulfill all the requirements of the body by keeping you healthy and fit.

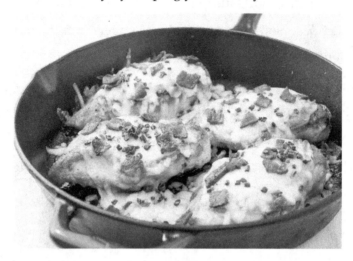

1. Creamy Tuscan garlic chicken

Servings: 6 | Total time: 25 min

Calories: 368 kcal | Proteins: 30 g | Carbohydrates: 7 g | Fat: 25 g

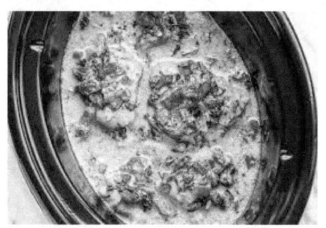

Ingredients

o   One and a half pounds of boneless chicken breasts

o   Two Tablespoons of olive oil

o   One cup cream

- o Half cup of chicken broth
- o One teaspoon of garlic powder
- o One teaspoon of italian seasoning
- o Half cup of parmesan cheese
- o One cup spinach chopped
- o Half cup tomatoes dried

Steps of preparation

- o Put olive oil in a wide skillet and cook chicken on medium-high heat for 3-5 minutes per side or until golden around each side and cook until the middle is no longer pink. Remove the chicken then put that aside on a tray.
- o Transfer some chicken broth, heavy cream, Italian seasoning, garlic powder, and parmesan cheese. Mix over medium-high heat unless it begins to thicken. Include the spinach and the sundried tomatoes and boil before the spinach starts wilting. Add the chicken to the skillet and, if needed, pour over pasta.
- o Serve with a lemon slice.

2. Avocado Greek salad

Servings: 4 | Total time: 15 min

Calories: 305 kcal | Proteins: 10 g | Carbohydrates: 12 g | Fat: 27 g

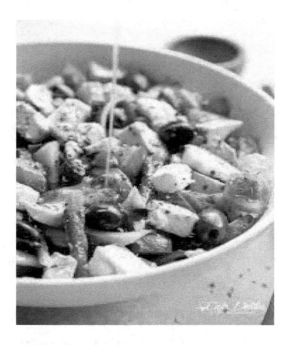

Ingredients

o   One by four cup olive oil

o   Two tablespoons vinegar

o   One teaspoon garlic paste

o   Two teaspoons dried oregano

o   One fourth teaspoon salt

o   One large sliced cucumber

o   Four wedge cut tomatoes

o   One green pepper sliced

o   Half sliced red onion

o   200 g cubed creamy feta cheese

o   Half cup olives

o   One large diced avocado

Steps of preparation

o   Mix together the spices of the dressing in the jar.

o   In a bowl, combine all the ingredients of the salad. Toss the dressing. Season with some salt only if required (depending about how salty your feta cheese is). Sprinkle on additional oregano to use. Start serving with chicken, lamb, beef, fish; the choices are infinite!

3. Keto Eggs and Zoodles

Servings: 2 | Total time: 25 min

Calories: 633 kcal | Proteins: 20 g | Carbohydrates: 27 g | Fat: 53 g

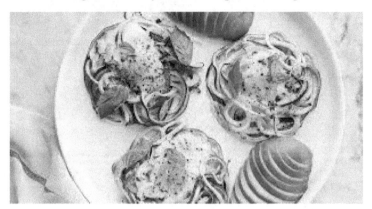

Ingredients

o   Nonstick spray

o   Three zucchinis

o   Two tablespoons olive oil

o   A pinch of Kosher salt and black pepper

o   Four large eggs

o   Red-pepper flakes

o   Basil

o   Two thinly sliced avocados

Steps of preparation

o   Preheat oven to 350 ° degrees F. Lightly oil a nonstick spray baking sheet.

o   In a wide pan, mix the zucchini noodles with the olive oil. Season to taste with the salt and the pepper. Divide into Four even parts, move to the baking tray, and build a nest shape.

o   steadily crack the egg in the center of each nest. Bake until eggs are ready, for 9 to 11 minutes. Season to taste with salt and pepper, garnish with red pepper flakes and basil. Serve with the slices of avocado.

4. Cheese and the Cauliflower 'Breadsticks

Servings: 4 | Total time: 20 min

Calories: 200 kcal | Proteins: 12 g | Carbohydrates: 9 g | Fat: 14 g

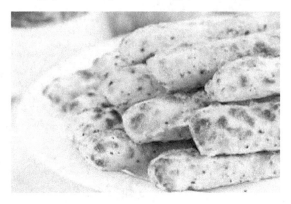

Ingredients

o   One head cauliflower

o   Two garlic cloves

o   One third cup mozzarella cheese

o   One third cup Parmesan cheese

o   Two eggs

o   One egg white

o   One tablespoon thyme

o   One tablespoon rosemary chopped

o   A pinch of Kosher salt and black pepper

o   Two tablespoons of olive oil

Steps of preparation

o   Begin by preheating the oven to a temperature of 425 ° F. Cover a baking sheet of parchment paper.

o   In a food processor bowl, mix the cauliflower with the garlic. Pulse until the finely chopped like a fine meal, for around three minutes. Move to a broad blending pot.

o   Mix the mozzarella, eggs, thyme, parmesan, egg white, and rosemary in the cauliflower until well blended; add salt and pepper.

- o Spread the cauliflower mixture in a 1/2-inch-thick ring upon the baking sheet. Brush the olive oil on the surface. Bake until the sides are crisp and light golden, for 25 to 30 minutes.
- o Cool for five min before cutting and able to serve in the sticks.

5. Rainbow Dinner Keto Chicken

Servings: 4 | Total time: 45 min

Calories: 394 kcal | Proteins: 39 g | Carbohydrates: 23 g | Fat: 16 g

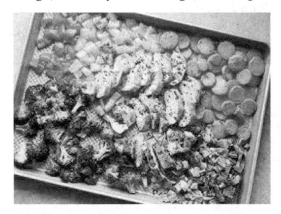

Ingredients

- o Nonstick spray
- o One-pound chicken
- o One tablespoon sesame oil
- o Two tablespoons soy sauce
- o Two tablespoons honey
- o Two diced red bell peppers
- o Two diced yellow bell peppers
- o Three sliced carrots
- o Half broccoli
- o Two diced red onions
- o Two tablespoons of olive oil
- o A pinch of Kosher salt and black pepper
- o One fourth cup chopped parsley

Steps of preparation

o Begin by Preheating the oven to a temperature of 400 ° F. Spray a baking sheet slightly with a nonstick spray.

o Put the chicken upon this baking sheet. In a bowl, shake with the sesame oil and the soy sauce. Brush the paste uniformly with the chicken.

o Place the red bell peppers, the yellow bell peppers, the vegetables, the broccoli, and the red onion on a baking sheet. Sprinkle the olive oil all over the vegetables and stir gently to coat, now season with some salt and pepper.

o Bake until the vegetables are soft as well as the chicken is thoroughly cooked for 23 to 25 minutes. Pull the mixture from oven and season with parsley.

6. Keto Dinner Chicken Meatballs

Servings: 4 | Total time: 45 min

Calories: 205 kcal | Proteins: 20 g | Carbohydrates: 3 g | Fat: 13 g

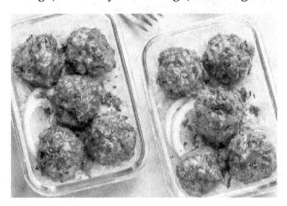

Ingredients

o One tablespoon olive oil

o Half chopped red onion

o 2 tablespoon minced garlic

o One-pound ground chicken

o One fourth cup chopped fresh parsley

o One tablespoon mustard paste

o Three fourth teaspoon kosher salt

o Half teaspoon black pepper

o One can coconut milk

- One and ¼ cups fresh parsley chopped
- Four chopped scallions
- One garlic minced
- One lemon zest and juice
- A pinch of Kosher salt and black pepper
- A pinch of Red pepper flakes
- One recipe Cauliflower Rice

Steps of preparation

- Start by Preheating the oven to 375 ° F. Lay a baking sheet with an aluminum foil and coat this with a non - stick cooking spray.
- Heat the olive oil in a medium skillet over medium heat. Include the onion and sauté until soft, for about five minutes. Include the garlic and sauté until fragrant for around 1 minute.
- Move the garlic and the onion to a medium bowl and let it cool moderately. Stir in parsley, chicken, and the mustard, sprinkle in pepper and salt. Shape the mixture into 2 tablespoon spheres and shift to the baking sheet.
- Bake the meatballs unless solid and thoroughly cooked for 17 to 20 mins.
- In a food processor jar, mix parsley, scallions, garlic, coconut milk, lemon zest, and lemon juice and mix thoroughly, sprinkle with salt and black pepper.
- Cover with both the red pepper flakes as well as the remaining parsley. Serve the sauce over cauliflower rice.

7. Keto Dinner Pork Carnitas

Servings: 4 | Total time: 45 min

Calories: 205 kcal | Proteins: 20 g | Carbohydrates: 3 g | Fat: 13 g

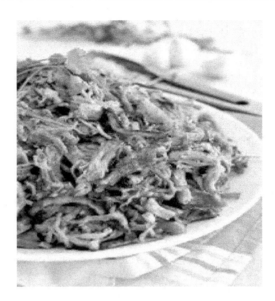

Ingredients

o One sliced white onion

o Five minced garlic cloves

o One minced jalapeño

o Three pounds pork shoulder (diced)

o A pinch of salt and black pepper

o One tablespoon cumin

o Two tablespoons fresh oregano

o Two oranges

o One lime

o One-third cup of chicken broth

Steps of preparation

o Put the onion, garlic, the jalapeno, and the pork at the bottom of the slow cooker. Put cinnamon, oregano pepper, and cumin to taste.

o Put the oranges and lime zest all over the pork, and then halve them and drop the juice all over the pork. Spill the broth over the pork as well.

o Place the cover on the slow cooker and hold the heat down. Cook for almost 7 hours or till meat is soft and quick to break with a fork.

o Utilize two forks to crumble the beef. Pork may be presented immediately (we like it in tacos) or frozen in an airtight jar in a refrigerator for up to 5 days or in a freezer for up to 1 month.

8. Keto Butter Scallops Garlic and Steak

Servings: 4 | Total time: 45 min

Calories: 205 kcal | Proteins: 20 g | Carbohydrates: 3 g | Fat: 13 g

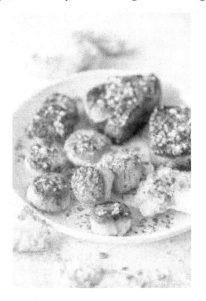

Ingredients

o Two beef tenderloin fillets

o A pinch of Kosher salt and black pepper

o Three tablespoons unsalted butter

o Eight to ten large sea scallops

o Three minced garlic cloves

o Six tablespoons cubed unsalted butter

o Two tablespoons parsley leaves chopped

o Two tablespoons fresh chives

o One tablespoon lemon juice

o Two teaspoons lemon zest

o A pinch of Kosher salt and black pepper

Steps of preparation

o Warm a cast iron pan on a medium-high flame for ten minutes.

o Use paper towels, pat all sides of steak dry; spice with some salt and pepper as you want.

o Melt 2 tbsp of butter. Put the steaks in the center of the pan and cook for around 4-6 mins until the thick crust has developed. Use tongs, flip and simmer for another five minutes or until done as desired; set the pan aside, cover it loosely.

o As the steak rests, clean the steak and heat the leftover one tablespoon of butter into it.

o Strip the short side muscle from of the scallops, clean with cold water, and dry completely.

o Season with salt and black pepper. Work in rounds, add the scallops to the pan in a single layer and fry, flip once, till golden brown and transparent in the middle, approximately three minutes per side. Put aside and leave it warm.

o Reducing overall heat to low for garlic butter sauce; add the garlic and simmer, stir constantly, until fragrant, for around 1 minute. Stir in butter, chives, lemon juice, parsley, and lemon zest, now season with salt and pepper.

o In the end, serve steaks and scallops directly with the garlic butter sauce.

9. Ketogenic Cauliflower Crispy Wrapped Prosciutto Bites

Servings: 8-10 | Total time: 45 min

Calories: 215 kcal | Proteins: 14 g | Carbohydrates: 5 g | Fat: 15 g

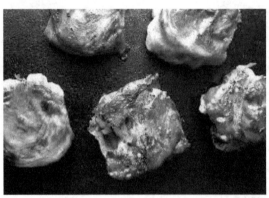

Ingredients

o One small head cauliflower

o Half cup tomato paste

o Two tablespoons white wine

o   Half teaspoon black pepper

o   Half cup grated Parmesan cheese

o   Twenty slices prosciutto

o   Six tablespoons olive oil

Steps of preparation

o   Cut the bottom of the cauliflower and some green leaves. Split the cauliflower in half and slice the half into one-inch-thick strips. Split the slices into two or three bits, based on the size of the slice.

o   Put to a boil a big pot of salted water. Blanch the cauliflower in water until it is almost soft, for 3 to 5 minutes. Remove the cauliflower and pat dry with the help of paper towels.

o   In a small cup, combine the tomato paste with black pepper and white wine. Layer 1 tsp along each side of the cauliflower, then top with 1 tsp of Parmesan. Gently seal a prosciutto slice over each piece of the cauliflower, gripping gently at the end to secure

o   Work in batches, cook two teaspoons of olive oil in a wide pan over medium heat. Bring the cauliflower then cook till the prosciutto is crispy and golden, three to four minutes per side. Then repeat with some extra oil and cauliflower until all the bits are fried. Let it settle slowly, then serve.

10. Ketogenic Fried Chicken Recipe

Servings: 12 | Total time: 12 min

Calories: 308 kcal | Proteins: 40.4 g | Carbohydrates: 0.7 g | Fat: 14 g

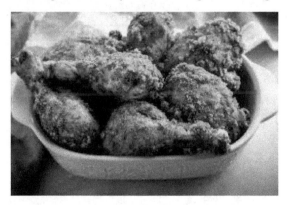

Ingredients

o   Four ounces of pork rinds

o   One and a half teaspoon thyme dried

o   One teaspoon sea salt dried

o   One teaspoon black pepper dried

o   One teaspoon oregano dried

o   Half teaspoon garlic powder dried

o   One teaspoon paprika dried

o   Twelve chicken legs and thighs

o   One egg

o   Two ounces mayonnaise

o   Three tablespoons of mustard

Steps of preparation

o   Start by preheating the oven at a temperature of 400 degrees Fahrenheit.

o   Grind pork rinds in a powder form, leaving them in a few bigger pieces.

o   Mix pork rinds with thyme, pepper, oregano, salt, garlic, and smoked paprika. Spread on a large plate into a thin sheet.

o   In a big container, mix egg, mayonnaise, and Dijon mustard. Dip every piece of chicken in the egg-mayonnaise mixture, and then wrap in the pork rind blend until it is thinly coated.

o   Put the chicken on a wire rack on a baking sheet and then bake for almost 40 minutes.

11. Greek Yogurt Chicken Peppers salad

Servings: 6 | Total time: 30 min

Calories: 116 kcal | Proteins: 7 g | Carbohydrates: 16 g | Fat: 3 g

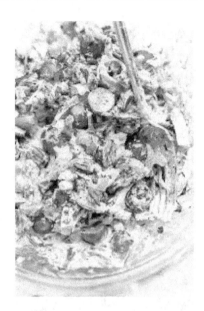

Ingredients

o   Two-third cup of Greek yogurt

o   Two tablespoons mustard paste

o   Two tablespoons vinegar

o   A pinch of Kosher salt and black pepper

o   One-third cup of chopped fresh parsley

o   Half kg of cubed roseate chicken

o   Two sliced stalks celery

o   One bunch of sliced scallions

o   One pint of cherry tomatoes

o   Half diced cucumber

o   Three bell peppers

Steps of preparation

o   In a bowl, combine Greek yogurt, and rice vinegar, and mustard; add salt and pepper. Put some parsley.

o   Include chicken, celery and three - fourths of the scallions, and cucumbers and tomatoes. Stir well and mix.

o   Distribute the chicken salad between the bell peppers.

o   Garnish the remainder scallions, some tomatoes, and cucumbers.

12. Easy chicken low carb stir fry recipe

Serving: 2 | Total Time: 12 mins

Calories: 219 | Fat:10g | Net Carbs:5.5g | Protein:19g

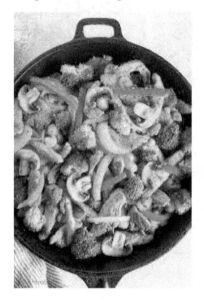

Ingredients

o   Sesame oil 1 tbsp

o   Boneless & skinless chicken thighs 2

o   Minced fresh ginger 1 Tbsp

o   Gluten-free soy sauce 1/4 cup

o   Water 1/2 cup

o   Onion powder 1 tsp

o   Garlic powder 1/2 tsp

o   Red pepper flakes 1 tsp

o   Granulated sugar1 Tbsp

o   Xanthan gum 1/2 tsp

o   Bagged broccolis mix 2 heaping cups

o   Chopped scallions 1/2 cup

Steps of Preparation

o Cut the chicken thighs into thin pieces/strips. Mix the chicken & chopped ginger in the edible oil in a big sauté pan for 2 to 3 mins.

o Apply the water, soy sauce, powder of onion, powder of garlic, red pepper flakes, sugar sub & xanthan gum. Remove well and simmer for five mins.

o Apply the slaw & scallions then coat – simmer for two min.

13. Keto Asiago Chicken with Bacon Cream Sauce

Serving: 4 | Total Time: 40 mins

Calories 581 kcal | Fat:38g | Net Carbs:8g | Protein:49g

Ingredients

o Chicken breasts 1.5 lb.

o Vegetable oil 1 1/2 tbsp

o Salt & pepper

o Minced garlic cloves 4

o Chicken stock 1 cup

o Cooked & chopped bacon 8 slices

o Sliced lemon 1/2

o Half & half 1 cup

o Shredded asiago cheese 1/2 cup

o Fresh chopped parsley 2 tbsp

Steps of Preparation

o Season the chicken nicely with salt & pepper on each side. Heat the vegetable fats in the big pan. Roast the chicken breasts over med-high heat-around two mins on per side to brown a bit. Do not cook the chicken thru-you will continue to cook it afterward. Take away the chicken from your Pan.

o Add chopped garlic to the same pan. Cook on med heat for around thirty sec, scraping the bottom of the skillet. Deglaze the skillet with a little chicken stock. Apply the leftover stock (total 1 cup).

o Apply half the bacon to the chicken broth.

- o Return the chicken to the saucepan, on top of the bacon, as well as in the broth of the chicken. Prepare 5 slim lemon slices across the breasts of the chicken and cook, boiling at low heat, covered for around twenty mins, till the chicken is fully cooked & no longer pink in the middle.

- o Take away the chicken from the pan after it is fully cooked. Remove the slices of lemon from the pan. It is much important to remove them. Do not abandon them in for the sauce, or else it'll be too sour. Put one half-and-a-half cup to the pan. Bring to the boil & stir well, scrap from the bottom. Apply 1/2 cup of Asiago shredded cheese & mix to melt totally, just around thirty sec.

- o Spoon a little sauce on the chicken breasts to serve & toss with the leftover minced bacon & minced parsley.

14. Ketogenic Grilled Chicken Souvlaki with Yogurt Sauce

Serving 4 | Total Time: 2hour 10 mins |

Calories: 192 | Fat:7g | Net Carbs:2.5g | Protein:27g

Ingredients

- o Chicken breast (cut in strips) 1 lb.
- o Olive oil 3 tbsp
- o Lemon juice 3 tbsp
- o Red wine vinegar 1 tbsp
- o Fresh chopped oregano 1 tbsp
- o Minced garlic 4 cloves
- o Kosher salt 2 tsp
- o Ground black pepper 1/4 tsp
- o Dried thyme 1/2 tsp

For the yogurt sauce

- o Greek yogurt 3/4 cup
- o Lemon juice 1 tsp
- o Minced Garlic 1 tsp
- o Fresh chopped oregano 1 tsp
- o Kosher salt 1/2 tsp

- o Granulated sugar 1/2 tsp

Steps of Preparation

- o In a small non-reactive bowl, mix the oil of olive, juice of lemon, red vinegar, garlic, oregano, pepper, salt, & dried thyme.
- o Fill the marinade with the chicken strips and combine well to cover.
- o Cover in the freezer & marinate for two hours or longer.
- o Take away the chicken from marinade & thread (when using) on skewers.
- o Heat the grill & grill the chicken for around two mins each side, or when it is cooked thru.

For the yogurt sauce:

- o Mix all the ingredients of the yogurt sauce & mix well. Season it with your preference.
- o Serve the hot grilled chicken with them.

15. Low Carb Chicken Jalapeño Poppers

Serving 15 | Total Time: 30 mins

Calories: 111 | Fat:9g | Net Carbs:1g | Protein:1g

Ingredients

- o Jalapenos large 15
- o Sharp shredded cheddar cheese 1 cup
- o Softened cream cheese 8 oz
- o Shredded & chopped cooked chicken 2 cups
- o Salsa Verde 1/3 cup
- o Garlic powder 1/2 tsp
- o Kosher salt 1/2 tsp
- o Cajun seasoning 1 tsp
- o Pulverized pork rinds 1 cup
- o Cajun seasoning 1/2 tsp

Steps of Preparation

- o Slice each pepper one/three off the top & scoop out in there.
- o Put the peppers on a tray & microwave to soften for two mins.

- In a med bowl, mix cream cheese, cheddar cheese, chicken/turkey, salsa Verde, powder of garlic, salt & Cajun seasoning, then mix till it's blended & creamy.
- Spoon the blend within the jalapeños.
- Mix the pork rind powder & Cajun seasoning in a tiny bowl.
- Nicely roll the cream cheese part of the filled jalapeños into the rinds of Cajun pork till covered.
- Put on the baking sheet.
- Cook for twenty mins at 400, or till its color changes to golden brown & bubble.
- Cool before serving, for a minimum of five mins.

16. Lemon butter chicken

Total Time: 50 mins | Serving: 8

Ingredients

- Chicken thighs 8 bone
- Smoked paprika 1 tbsp
- Ground black pepper & kosher salt
- Divided unsalted butter 3 tbsp
- Minced garlic 3 cloves
- Chicken broth 1 cup
- Heavy cream 1/2 cup
- Freshly grated parmesan 1/4 cup
- Lemon juice 1
- Dried thyme 1 tsp
- Chopped baby spinach 2 cups

Steps of Preparation

- Oven Preheated to 205 degrees C.
- Top chicken thighs with salt, paprika & pepper.
- Melt two tbsp of butter on med-high heat in a big oven-proof pan. Put chicken, skin side down, & sear on each side till they become golden brown, approximately 2 to 3 mins each side; sink excess fat & set it aside.

- o Melt the remaining tbsp of butter in the pan. Apply the garlic & cook till fragrant, constantly whisking, approximately 1 to 2 mins, mix in chicken broth, whipping cream, parmesan, juice of lemon, and thyme.
- o Bring to a boil; lower the heat, mix in the spinach & boil till the spinach had also wilted & the sauce had already thickened slightly around 3 to 5 mins.
- o Put in the oven & roast for around 25 to 30 min till fully cooked, trying to reach a core temp of 75 degrees C.
- o Serve asap.

17. Keto Chicken Low Carb Stir Fry.

Servings: 4 | Total time: 22 min

Calories: 116 kcal | Proteins: 28 g | Carbohydrates: 9 g | Fat: 7 g

Ingredients

- o One fourth Olive oil
- o One-pound Chicken breast
- o Half teaspoon sea salt
- o One by four teaspoon Black pepper
- o Four Garlic minced
- o Six ounces of Broccoli
- o One Red bell pepper
- o One fourth cup Chicken bone broth
- o One-pound Cauliflower rice
- o One fourth Coconut aminos
- o One teaspoon Toasted sesame oil
- o One fourth cup green onions

Steps of preparation

o Heat 2 tablespoons of olive oil in a large pan over medium heat. Include the strips of chicken and add salt and pepper. Now cook for 4-5 minutes, turning once, until chicken is crispy and just cooked thru.

o Remove the chicken from the pan, set it aside, then cover to keep it warm.

o Apply the remaining two tbsp (30 ml) of olive oil in a pan. Include the crushed garlic and then sauté for around a minute until aromatic.

o Include the broccoli and the bell pepper. Cook for 3-4 minutes before the broccoli begins to turn bright green, and the peppers tend to soften.

o Add the broth of bone. To deglaze, scrape the base of the pan. Reduce to medium temperature. Cover the pan and simmer for 3-5 minutes, until the broccoli is crisp.

o Transfer coconut aminos to pan, scrape the bottom of the pan and deglaze again. Put the chicken back in the pan. Transfer the rice to the cauliflower. Heat up to medium-high again. Now Stir for 3-4 minutes, before the cauliflower is tender but not mushy, most liquid evaporates, and the chicken is fully cooked through.

o Remove from the heat. Cover in toasted sesame oil. Add salt and black pepper if necessary. Cover with green onion, as needed

18. Keto Tomato chicken zoodles

Servings: 4 | Total time: 20 min

Calories: 411 kcal | Proteins: 45 g | Carbohydrates: 11 g | Fat: 18.8 g

Ingredients

o Coconut butter ½ tsp

o Diced onion 1 medium

o Chicken fillets 450- 500 g

o Garlic clove, 1 minced

o Zucchinis two medium

o Crushed tomatoes 400 g

o Chop half 7-10 cherry tomatoes

o Cashews 100 g

o Salt

- Dry oregano & basil
- Black pepper

Steps of preparation

- Heat a wide pan over medium heat. Add the coconut butter and the sliced onion. Cook for about 30 seconds to about 1 minute. Be alert, so you don't roast the onions.
- Slice the chicken into 2 cm chunks.
- Apply chicken and garlic to the pan. Season with the basil, the oregano salt and black pepper. Cook the chicken for about 5-6 minutes each side.
- Spiralize the zucchini when the chicken is frying. Cut them short when they're wanted. Use the vegetable peeler to create the ribbons out from the zucchini.
- Add the crushed tomatoes and simmer for about 3-5 minutes.
- Cook the cashews in another pan until golden brown. Taste and adjust with paprika, some turmeric and salt.
- Now add the spiralled zoodles, some cherry tomatoes and sprinkle with extra salt as appropriate. Cook for the next 1 minute and then switch off the heat.
- Now serve chicken zoodles with crispy cashews and the fresh basil.

19. Tuscan garlic chicken

Servings: 6 | Total time: 25 min

Calories: 225 kcal | Proteins: 30 g | Carbohydrates: 7 g | Fat: 25 g

Ingredients

- *Boneless chicken breasts 1½ pounds*
- *Olive oil 2 Tablespoons*
- *Heavy cream 1 cup*
- *Chicken broth 1/2 cup*
- *Garlic powder 1 teaspoon*
- *Italian seasoning 1 teaspoon*
- *Parmesan cheese 1/2 cup*
- *Chopped spinach 1 cup*
- *Dried tomatoes 1/2 cup*

Steps of Preparation

o   Put olive oil in a wide skillet and cook chicken on medium heat for about 3-5 minutes on every side or until it gets brown on each side and then cook until the middle is no longer pink. Remove the chicken and put it aside on a tray.

o   Include some of the chicken broth, the garlic powder, the heavy cream, the Italian seasoning and also some parmesan cheese. Simmer over on a medium-high flame until it thickens. Include the spinach and the tomatoes and then cook before the spinach becomes soggy. Transfer the chicken onto the plate.

o   Serve over pasta.

20. Turkey and peppers

Servings: 4 | Total time: 20 min

Calories: 230 kcal | Proteins: 30 g | Carbohydrates: 11 g | Fat: 8 g

Ingredients

o   Salt 1 teaspoon

o   Turkey tenderloin 1 pound

o   Olive oil 2 tablespoons

o   Sliced onion ½ large

o   Red bell pepper 1

o   Yellow bell pepper 1

o   Italian seasoning ½ teaspoon

o   Black pepper ¼ teaspoon

o   Vinegar 2 teaspoons

o   Crushed tomatoes 14-ounce

o   Parsley and basil for garnishing

Steps of preparation

o   Sprinkle outa 1/2 teaspoon of salt over the turkey. Heat 1 tablespoon of the oil in a wide non-stick pan over medium heat. Include almost half of the turkey and then cook until golden brown on the rim, for 1 to 3 minutes. Flip and continue to cook for 2 minutes. Now remove the turkey from the slotted spatula to the tray, cover with foil to keep it warm. Apply the remaining 1 tablespoon of oil to the pan, reduce the heat to low and then repeat with the remaining turkey for 1 to 3 minutes per side.

o Transfer the onion, the bell peppers and the remainder 1/2 teaspoon of the salt to the pan, cover and simmer, then remove the lid and stir often, until the onion and the peppers are softened and golden brown in the spots for almost 5 to 7 minutes.

o Replace the cover, raise the heat to almost medium-high, then sprinkle with Italian seasoning and pepper and roast with stirring constantly before the herbs are fragrant for around 30 seconds. Now add vinegar and then cook until almost fully evaporated, for around 20 seconds. Put tomatoes and bring to a simmer, stirring regularly.

o Transfer the turkey to the pan with any leftover juices and bring to simmer. Now reduce the heat to medium-low and then cook until the turkey is hot all through the sauce for almost 1 to 2 minutes. Serve topped with parsley and basil if it's used.

21. Ketogenic Ginger butter chicken

Servings: 4 | Total time: 20 min

Calories: 293 kcal | Proteins: 29 g | Carbohydrates: 9 g | Fat: 17 g

Ingredients

o Cubed chicken breast 1.5 pounds

o Garam masala 2 tablespoons

o Fresh ginger grated 3 teaspoons

o Minced garlic 3 teaspoons

o Greek yogurt 4 ounces

o Coconut oil 1 tablespoon

o Ghee 2 tablespoons

o Onion sliced 1

o Fresh ginger grated 2 teaspoons

o Minced garlic 2 teaspoons

o Can crushed tomatoes 14.5 oz

o Ground coriander 1 tablespoon

o Garam masala ½ tablespoon

o   Cumin 2 teaspoons

o   Chili powder 1 teaspoon

o   Heavy cream ½ cup

o   Salt

o   Cilantro

Instruction

O   Slice chicken into 2 inches pieces and put in a wide bowl with 2 teaspoons of garam masala, one teaspoon of fried ginger and one teaspoon of minced garlic. Attach the yogurt, whisk to mix. Transfer to the refrigerator and cool for at least 30 minutes.

O   Place the onion, ginger, garlic, and spices and crushed tomatoes in a blender and blend until soft. Set it aside

O   Heat 1 tablespoon oil in a wide pan over medium heat. Put chicken and marinade in the pan, fry three to four minutes per side. After browning, add in the sauce and simmer for 5 to 6 minutes.

O   Mix in the heavy cream and ghee and proceed to cook for another minute. Taste the salt and apply the extra if necessary. Cover with cilantro and, if needed, serve with some cauliflower rice.

22. Keto BLT Lettuce Wraps

Total Time: 25 minutes | Servings: 4

Calories: Kcal 368 | Fat: 30.8g | Net Carbs: 15.8g | Protein: 11.6g

Ingredients

o   From 1 med head butter lettuce 8 leaves, like Bibb or Boston

o   Bacon 6 slices

o   Mayonnaise 2 tbsp

o   Fine chopped chives 1 tbsp

o   Squeezed freshly lemon juice 1 tbsp

o   Black pepper ground freshly 1/8 tsp

o   Grape tomatoes half or pint cherry 1

o   Diced avocado 1 med

Steps of Preparation

o   Set up a rack in the bottom third of the oven and to 400 ° F heat it. Lined a baking sheet with an aluminum foil or parchment paper.

o   Place the bacon in one layer onto the baking sheet. Bake 15 to 20 mins until crispy and rich golden-brown. From the oven, Remove and allow cool. Alternatively, in a shallow pot, mix the mayonnaise, lemon juice, chives, and pepper; set aside.

o   Move the bacon to a cutting board until it's cold and chop it roughly. Load a single leaf of lettuce with tomatoes, avocado, and bacon. Drizzle with the dressing, then serve.

23. Chipotle Avocado Mayonnaise

Total Time: 5 minutes | Serving 1

Calories Kcal 188| Fat: 18.9g |Net Carbs: 5.8g| Protein: 1.4g

Ingredients

o   Medium avocados 2 ripe

o   Chipotle chile canned finely chopped in adobo sauce 1 tsp

o   Dijon mustard 1 tsp

o   Lemon juice freshly squeezed 1 tsp

o   Kosher salt 1/2 tsp

o   Olive oil 1/4 cup

Steps of Preparation

o   In a mini food processor or blender, place the chipotle chili, avocados, in adobo sauce, lemon juice, Dijon mustard, and kosher salt. Process till smooth, for 30 - 1 minute. Scrape the bowl or pitcher side. Switch on the machine and drizzle gradually into the oil. Blend, about 1 minute, till smooth & emulsified.

24. Keto Egg Dinner Muffins

Total Time:15 minutes | Serving 12 muffins

Calories: Kcal 227 | Fat: 7.3g | Net Carbs: 5.3g| Protein: 11.7g

Ingredients

o   Olive oil or Cooking spray

o   Sweet potato shredded 1 1/2 cups

o   Cheddar cheese shredded sharp 1 cup

o   Strips bacon sugar-free, crumbled 6 cooked

o   Large eggs 10

o   Kosher salt 1 teaspoon

o   Black pepper freshly ground 1/4 tsp

Steps of Preparation

o   Arrange a middle-rack in -oven and to 400 ° F heat. Coat a regular 12 well muffin tray generously with olive oil or cooking spray. Divide the sliced sweet potato, bacon, and cheese equally throughout the wells of muffins.

o   In a big cup, put the eggs, half-&-a-half, pepper, and salt and whisk till the eggs are thoroughly integrated. Pour in the wells of the muffins, filling 1/2 to 3/4 complete each.

o   Bake for 12 - 14 minutes, till the muffins, are set and brown slightly around edges. On a wire rack, place the pan and allow it to cool for 2 - 3 mins. Run the butter knife to the release of the muffins around cups each of them before extracting them. Serve cold or warm, before cooling or freezing, absolutely on a wire rack.

25. Prosciutto-Wrapped Avocado with Arugula and Goat Cheese

Total Time: 15 minutes | Servings 4

Calories: Kcal 295 | Fat: 23.1 | Net Carbs: 9.6g | Protein: 15.4g

Ingredients

o   Goat cheese fresh 4 ounces

o   Lemon juice freshly squeezed 2 tbsp

o   Black pepper freshly ground 1/2 tsp

o   Kosher salt 1/4 tsp

o   Prosciutto 8 thin slices

o   Arugula 1 1/2 cups

o   Thinly sliced avocados ripe medium 2

Steps of Preparation

o In a shallow pot, mix the goat cheese, lemon juice, salt, and pepper until smooth. Place pieces of the prosciutto. Layer single slice of prosciutto with 2 - 3 tsp of goat cheese mixture. Split the arugula into the prosciutto, placing the greens on one end of each piece. Cover each pile of greens similarly with 2–3 slices of avocado. Operating with one prosciutto slice at a time, then wrapping up into a compact package beginning with the avocado from the end.

26. Garlic Butter Steak Bites

Total Time: 20 minutes | Serving: 2-4

Calories: Kcal 748 | Fat: 61.9g | Net Carbs: 1.4g | Protein: 44.4g

Ingredients

o Garlic 4 cloves

o Black pepper freshly ground 1/2 teaspoon

o Parsley leaves chopped fresh 1/4 cup

o Thick-cut strip steaks New York 2 pounds

o Kosher salt 1/2 teaspoon

o Unsalted butter 8 tablespoons

Steps of Preparation

o Mince 4 cloves of garlic. Place in a cup and apply 1/2 tsp of black pepper freshly ground. Cut until 1/4 cup of fresh parsley leaves is available, then move to a small pot. Cut 2 pounds of strip steak New York into 1-inch pieces, then apply 1/2 tsp of kosher salt to season.

o Melt 8 tbsp (1 stick) of unsalted butter over medium-high heat in a large skillet. Attach the steak cubes then sear till browned, tossing them halfway through, taking 6 - 8 mins. Add the pepper and garlic, and simmer for another 1 minute. Take off the heat and with the parsley garnish.

27. Pesto Chicken with Burst Cherry Tomatoes

Total Time: 25-30 minutes | Serving 4

Calories: Kcal 445 | Fat: 16.2g | Net Carbs: 8.2g | Protein: 63.6g

Ingredients

o Grape tomatoes or pints cherry 2

o   Olive oil 1 tbsp

o   Kosher salt 1/2 tsp

o   Black pepper freshly ground 1/4 tsp

o   Chicken breasts boneless, skinless 4

o   Basil pesto 1/4 cup

Steps of Preparation

o   Place a rack in the center of the oven and to 400 ° F heat the oven.

o   Put the tomatoes on a baking sheet, which is rimmed. Remove the grease, season with pepper and salt, and mix. Spread out over a single sheet.

o   Pat, the chicken, completely dries it with paper towels. Season with pepper and salt. Put the chicken on the baking sheet in the middle. Spread the pesto on each chicken breast (about 1 tbsp each), spread on a thin layer, so each breast is covered evenly and fully.

o   Roast until caramelized the tomatoes have, and others have burst and cooked the chicken and registers 165 ° F, 25 - 30 mins, on a thermometer. Serve the drizzled chicken and tomatoes with pan juices.

28. Scrambled eggs with basil and butter

Total Time: 10 mins | Serving 1

Calories: Kcal 641 | Fat:59g | Net Carbs:3g | Protein:26g

Ingredients

o   Butter 2 tbsp

o   Eggs 2

o   Heavy whipping cream 2 tbsp

o   Ground black pepper & salt

o   Shredded cheese 2 oz

o   Fresh basil 2 tbsp

Steps of Preparation

o   Melt butter over low heat in a saucepan.

- o In a small cup, put cracked eggs, shredded cheese, cream, and seasoning. Offer it a quick whisk and apply it to the saucepan.
- o Push from the side to the middle with a spatula before the eggs are scrambled. If you want fluffy and soft, mix on lower heat to desired consistency.

29. Keto seafood special omelet

Total Time: 20 mins | Serving 2

Calories: Kcal 872 | Fat:83g | Net Carbs:4g | Protein:27g

Ingredients

- o Olive oil 2 tbsp
- o Cooked shrimp 5 oz
- o Red chili pepper 1
- o ½ tsp fennel seeds or ground cumin
- o Mayonnaise ½ cup
- o Fresh chives 1 tbsp
- o Eggs 6
- o Olive oil 2 tbsp
- o Salt & pepper

Steps of Preparation

- o Preheat the broiler.
- o In olive oil, broil the seafood or shrimp mixture with the chopped garlic, chili, cumin, fennel seeds, salt & pepper.
- o To cooled seafood mixture, apply mayo and chives.
- o Whisk the eggs together, season with salt & pepper, and cook in a non-stick saucepan with butter or oil.
- o When the omelet is nearly full, apply the seafood mixture. Fold. Reduce the heat and enable it to set fully. Serve.

30. Keto Fried eggs

Total Time: 10 mins | Serving 4

Per serving: Kcal 226, Fat:20g, Net Carbs:1g Protein:11g

Ingredients

o Butter 4 tbsp

o Eggs 8

o Salt & pepper

Steps of Preparation

o Heat coconut oil or butter over medium heat in a frying pan.

o Break the eggs directly into the saucepan. For sunny side up eggs, allow the eggs to be fried on one side. Cover the saucepan with a lid to ensure that they are fried on top. For eggs that are easily cooked, turn over the eggs after a few mins and then cook for another.

o Season with salt & pepper.

31. Keto egg butter with smoked salmon and avocado

Total Time: 20 mins |Serving 2

Calories: 1148, Fat:112g, Net Carbs:5g Protein:26g

Ingredients

o Eggs 4

o Sea salt ½ tsp

o Ground black pepper ¼ tsp

o Butter 5 oz

o Avocados 2

o Olive oil 2 tbsp

o Chopped fresh parsley 1 tbsp

o Smoked salmon 4 oz

Steps of Preparation

o Carefully put the eggs in a pot. Cover with colder water and place without the lid on the stove. Get the water to boil.

o Reduce heat and allow to simmer for 7-8 mins, from the warmed water. Remove the eggs and put them in an ice-cold bowl to cool.

- Peel and chop the eggs completely. Combine the eggs with the butter with the fork. Season with the pepper, salt, and other spices of your choosing
- Serve.

32. Ketogenic scallions egg muffins

Total Time: 25 mins | Serving 6

Calories: Kcal 336, Fat:26g, Net Carbs:2g Protein:23g

Ingredients

- Finely chopped scallions 2
- Chopped air-dried chorizo 5 oz.
- Eggs 12
- Salt & pepper
- Shredded cheese 6 oz

Steps of Preparation

- Preheat an oven to 175 ° C (350 ° F).
- Line a non-stick muffin tray with insertable baking cups/grease, a buttered silicone muffin tin.
- Apply the chorizo and scallions to the tin base.
- Mix the eggs with the pesto, pepper, and salt then incorporate the cheese and mix.
- Pour the batter over the scallions and the chorizo.
- Bake the muffin tin for 15–20 mins, depending on the scale.

33. Keto fried eggs with kale and pork

Total Time:20 mins | Serving 2

Calories: Kcal 1033, Fat:99g, Net Carbs:8g Protein:26g

Ingredients

- Kale ½ lb.
- Butter 3 oz
- Smoked pork belly 6 oz
- Frozen cranberries 1 oz
- Pecans 1 oz.

o Eggs 4

o Salt & pepper

Steps of Preparation

o Chop and Trim the kale into wide squares. Melt 2/3rd of the butter in the frying pan and cook the kale rapidly over high heat until the sides are slightly browned.

o From the frying pan, Remove the kale and put aside. Cook the bacon or pork belly in the frying pan until it is crisp.

o Reduce heat. The sautéed kale is Returned to the saucepan and add the nuts and cranberries. Remove until soft

o Turn the flame on the rest of the butter and fry the eggs. Add Salt and pepper. Put two fried eggs for each part of the greens and serve.

34. Keto Croque Monsieur

Total Time: 20 mins | Serving 2

Calories: Kcal 1083, Fat:92g, Net Carbs:8g Protein:54g

Ingredients

o Cottage cheese 8 oz

o Eggs 4

o Husk powder ground psyllium 1 tbsp

o Butter 4 tbsp

o deli ham 51/3 oz

o Cheddar cheese 51/3 oz

o Lettuce 3½ oz.

o Olive oil 4 tbsp

o Red wine vinegar ½ tbsp

o Salt & pepper

Steps of Preparation

- In a bowl, whisk the eggs. Blend in cottage cheese. Apply a psyllium husk powder ground when stirring in order incorporate it without lumps smoothly. Rest the mixture for five minutes before the batter has formed.
- Put the frying pan over med heat. Apply a large quantity of butter and cook the batter like tiny pancakes on either side for a few minutes, until they are brown.
- Create a sandwich between the two warm pancakes with cheese and sliced ham. Add finely diced onion on top.
- Wash and cut the lettuce. In a clear vinaigrette, add the oil, vinegar, salt, and pepper.

35. Veggie keto scramble

Total Time: 20 mins | Serving 1

Calories: Kcal 415, Fat:31g, Net Carbs:4g Protein:28g

Ingredients

- Butter 1 tbsp
- Sliced mushrooms 1 oz.
- Eggs 3
- Diced red bell peppers 1 oz
- Ground black pepper & salt
- Shredded parmesan cheese 1 oz
- Chopped scallion ½

Steps of Preparation

- Heat the butter over medium heat in a wide frying pan. Add the sliced mushrooms, diced red peppers, salt, and fry until tender.
- Put the eggs directly into the saucepan and quickly mix so that it is properly incorporated.
- Transfer the spatula to create big, soft curds over the bottom and side of the skillet. Cook until no clear liquid egg remains.
- Put the scramble with scallions and shredded parmesan on top.

36. Keto dinner chaffles

Time: 25 mins | Serving 4

Calories: Kcal 599, Fat:50g, Net Carbs:4g Protein:32g

Ingredients

- o Eggs 4
- o Shredded cheddar cheese 8 oz
- o Chopped fresh chives 2 tbsp
- o Salt & pepper

Toppings

- o Eggs 4
- o Sliced bacon 8
- o Sliced cherry tomatoes 8
- o Baby spinach 2 oz

Steps of Preparation

- o Heat the waffle maker.
- o Place the bacon slices in a big, unheated frying pan and raise the temperature to med heat. Cook the bacon for around 8-12 mins, regularly rotating, until it is crispy to taste.
- o Set aside to cool as you cook the chaffles on a paper towel.
- o Put all ingredients of your waffle in a mixing bowl & beat to blend.
- o Grind the waffle iron lightly and spoon the mixture equally over the bottom surface, spreading it out to achieve an even outcome.
- o Shut the waffle iron then cook according to the waffle maker for approx. 6 mins.
- o Break the eggs in the bacon grease in the frying pan as the chaffles are heating, then cook softly until finished.
- o Serve with scrambled egg and baby spinach, bacon strips, and cherry tomatoes on each chaffles side.

Chapter 5: Keto snacks recipes for women above 50

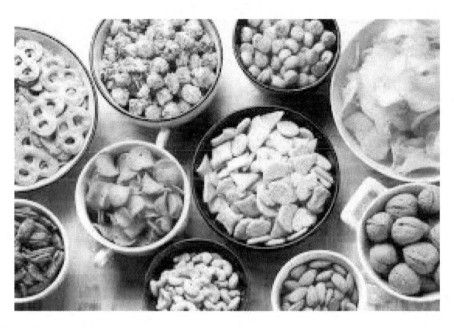

1. Keto Tortilla Chips

Servings: 10 chips | Total time: 40 min

Calories: 198 kcal | Proteins: 11 g | Carbohydrates: 4 g | Fat: 16 g

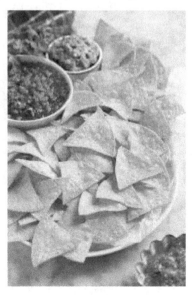

Ingredients

o   shredded mozzarella 2 cups

- o almond flour 1 cups
- o kosher salt 1 teaspoon
- o garlic powder 1 teaspoon
- o chili powder half teaspoon
- o Black pepper

Steps of preparation

- o Preheat the oven to 350 ° F. Place two big baking sheets of parchment paper.
- o Melt mozzarella in a microwave safe jar, around 1 minute and 30 seconds. Include almond flour, cinnamon, garlic powder, chili powder and several cracks of black pepper. Use your hands to knead the dough a few times until the ball is smooth.
- o Put the dough between the two sheets of the parchment paper and then roll it into a rectangle 1/8 "wide. Break the dough into triangles by using a knife.
- o Scatter the chips on the lined baking sheets and cook until the sides are crispy and begin to be crisp, for 12 to 14 minutes.

2. Ketogenic Avocado Chips

Servings: 6 chips | Total time: 30 min

Calories: 171 kcal | Proteins: 7 g | Carbohydrates: 6 g | Fat: 16 g

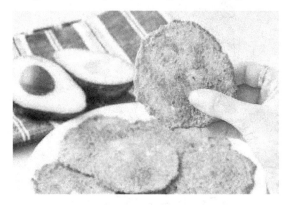

Ingredients

- o Ripe avocado 1 large
- o Freshly grated parmesan 3/4 cup.
- o Lemon juice 1 teaspoon
- o Garlic powder half teaspoon

o   Italian seasoning half teaspoon

o   A pinch of kosher salt

o   Black pepper

Steps of preparation

o   Start by Preheating the oven to 325 ° f and then line two baking sheets with a parchment paper. In a medium dish, mash the avocado with a fork until it is smooth. Stir in Parmesan, some lemon juice, some garlic powder and also Italian seasonings. Season with salt and pepper.

o   Put the heaping teaspoon-sized mixture scoops on the baking sheet, leaving around 3 "apart across each scoop. Deflate each scoop to 3 "wide with the wooden spoon or a cup. Now bake it until it is crispy and golden, for about 30 minutes, then let it cool to room temperature. Serve at room temperature.

o

3. Ketogenic Nacho Cheese Crisps

Servings: 9 chips | Total time: 1 hr. min

Calories:99   kcal | Proteins: 6 g | Carbohydrates:1.3 g | Fat: 7 g

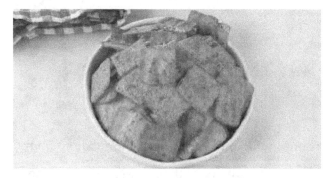

Ingredients

o   Sliced cheddar 8-oz.

o   Taco seasoning 2 tsp.

Steps of preparation

o   Start by preheating the oven to 250° and then line a baking sheet with a parchment paper. Now cut slices of cheese into about 9 squares and then place them in a medium bowl. Now add the taco seasoning.

o Put cheese slices on the prepared baking sheet. Now bake them until crisp and golden brown, for about 40 minutes. Let them cool for 10 minutes and then remove from the parchment paper.

4. Ketogenic coconut vanilla Ice Cream

Servings: 3　|　Total time: 10 min

Calories:　347 kcal | Proteins: 2 g | Carbohydrates: 3 g | Fat: 36 g

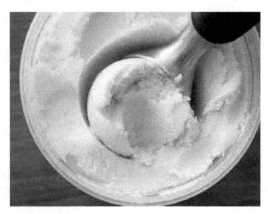

Ingredients

o Coconut milk 15-oz.

o Heavy cream 2 cup

o Swerve sweetener 1/4 cup

o Vanilla extract 1 tsp.

o A Pinch of kosher salt

Steps of preparation

o Start by chilling the coconut milk in the refrigerator for about 3 hours, preferably overnight.

o place the coconut cream in a big tub, leave the liquid in a can, using a hand blender to beat the coconut cream till it is very smooth. Set it back.

o Beat heavy cream in a separate wide bowl using a hand blender (or a stand mixer in a bowl) until soft peaks are created. Beat the sweetener and the vanilla.

o Fold the mixed coconut into the whipped cream, then move the mixture to the loaf tray.

o Freeze to a solid condition, around 5 hours.

5. Jalapeno popping Egg Cups

Servings: 12 cups　|　Total time: 45 min

Calories: 157 kcal | Proteins: 9.7 g | Carbohydrates: 1.3 g | Fat: 9.7 g

Ingredients

o   bacon 12 slices

o   large eggs 10

o   sour cream 1/4 c.

o   shredded cheddar half c.

o   shredded mozzarella half c.

o   sliced 2 jalapeños

o   a pinch of kosher salt

o   black pepper

o   cooking spray

Steps of preparation

o   Start by preheating the oven to 375° F. Cook bacon till it becomes slightly browned in a large pan over a medium flame, to drain, set it aside on a plate lined with paper towel.

o   In a separate bowl, mix the eggs together with cheeses, minced jalapeño, sour cream, and garlic powder. Now season with salt and pepper.

o   Grease a muffin tin through nonstick cooking spray. Put a slice of bacon and line each well, put egg mixture into every muffin cup. Garnish each muffin with a jalapeño slice.

o   Now bake for almost 20 minutes, or till the eggs are no longer looking wet. Now Cool them slightly.

o   Remove from the muffin tin and serve.

6. Ketogenic Bacon Guac Bombs

Servings: 1 | Total time: 45 min

Calories: 156 kcal | Proteins: 3.4 g | Carbohydrates: 1.4 g | Fat:15.2 g

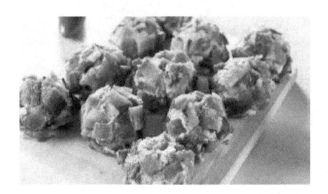

Ingredients

- o   cooked 12 slices bacon
- o   mashed 2 avocados
- o   cream cheese 6 oz.
- o   1 lime Juice
- o   minced garlic 1 clove
- o   minced 1/4 red onion
- o   jalapeno chopped 1 small
- o   cumin half tsp.
- o   Chili powder half tsp.
- o   A pinch of Kosher salt
- o   black pepper

Steps of preparation

- o   In a large bowl, put all the ingredients of the guacamole. Stir until it is mostly smooth and then season with the salt and pepper. Put gently in the refrigerator for almost 30 minutes.
- o   Put the crumbling bacon on a wide tray. Scoop the guacamole mixture with a little cookie scoop and put in the bacon. Roll to coat the bacon. Repeat before both guacamole and bacon are used. Store in the freezer.

7. Ketogenic TPW White Choc Truffles

Servings: 1 | Total time: 1 hour 15 min

Calories: 102 Kcal, | Fat: 7g | Protein: 7g | Carbohydrates: 3g

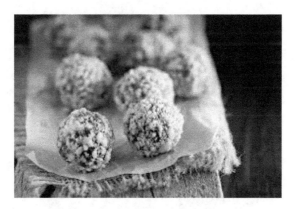

Ingredients

o Pea Protein 60g

o Chocolate Fudge 80g

o Syrup Honey flavor 10g

o dark chocolate 100g

o chopped salted peanuts 70g

Steps of preparation

o Mix the pea protein 80, the honey and the stuffed nuts in a wide bowl until mixed. If the mixture is too dry, apply some peanut butter. Apply more protein powder if the combination is too sticky.

o When your mixture is the consistency, you can accommodate, roll it into equal-sized balls (as large or small as you choose) and put it on a cling film or baking tray that is parchment lined. Refrigerate for an hour.

o When they're chilling, start to melt the chocolate in a heat-resistant container, either in a microwave or in a glass bowl over a boiling water pan.

o When melted, allow to cool moderately and cover with a cling film or with a baking sheet.

o Take the balls from the refrigerator and use a skewer coat in dark chocolate until each ball it is fully coated.

o Return to a baking tray and then sprinkle each truffle with salted chopped peanuts until coated.

o Return to the refrigerator for at least an hour to rest before dining.

o Remove and let it rest for a minute or two until you feed. Enjoy!

8. Brownie Fat Bombs

Servings: 1 | Total time: 45 min

Calories 118 Kcal | Carbs: 2g |Protein: 5g |Fat: 9g

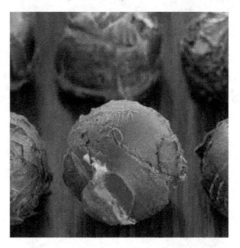

Ingredients

o   Smooth peanut butter 250g

o   Cocoa 65g

o   Zero syrup 2-4 tbsp

o   Coconut oil 2 tbsp

o   Salt ¼ tsp

Steps of preparation

o   Simply transfer all the ingredients to the food processor, rubbing near the bottom, if necessary, until mixed into a dough.

o   While using liquid sweetener or Zero Syrup or a coconut oil, refrigerate dough in refrigerator till the mixture is solid enough to scoop into a little scoop or spoonful of ice cream. Roll in the balls of your perfect size and serve and enjoy!

9. Cheesy Stuffed Mushrooms

Servings: 12 | Total time: 15 min

Calories: 72 Kcal, |Fat: 7g |Protein: 6g | Carbohydrates: 0g Fat: 5g

Ingredients

o   Bacon 225g

- o Mushrooms 12
- o Butter 2 tbsp
- o Cream cheese 200g
- o Finely chopped 3 tbsp chives,
- o Paprika powder 1 tsp
- o Salt and pepper

Steps of preparation

- o Start by preheating the oven to 200 ° F.
- o Now fry the bacon until it becomes really crisp. Enable to cool and afterward toss into the crumbs – save the fat of the bacon.
- o Take the stems from the shrooms and cut them finely. Fry in the bacon fat, add the butter if needed.
- o In a dish, blend the bacon crumbs with the fried mushroom stems and the leftover marinade.
- o Cover each of the mushrooms with a mixture and then bake for 20 minutes until it gets golden brown.

10. Keto Peanut Butter Granola

Servings: 12 | Total time: 40 min

Calories: 338 Kcal, | Fat: 30g | Protein: 9g | Carbohydrates: 9g

Ingredients

- o Almonds 1 1/2 cups
- o Pecans 1 1/2 cups
- o Coconut 1 cup shredded
- o Sunflower seeds 1/4 cup
- o Swerve Sweetener 1/3 cup
- o Vanilla 1/3 cup
- o Peanut butter 1/3 cup
- o Butter 1/4 cup
- o Water 1/4 cup

Steps of preparation

o   Preheat the oven to 300F and line a wide-rimmed baking tray with a parchment paper.

o   Process the almonds and pecans in a processor until they match rough crumbs with some bigger parts. Now transfer them to a large bowl and then mix in a, sunflower seeds, shredded coconut, sweetener and some vanilla extract.

o   Now melt the peanut butter and the butter together in a microwave safe jar.

o   Pour the molten peanut butter mixture over the nut mixture and combine gently, stirring gently. Stir it in the water. Mixture is going to clump together.

o   Now spread mixture uniformly on the prepared lined baking sheet for 30 minutes, by stirring halfway through. Now remove and let it cool off completely.

11. Ketogenic hot caramel chocolate

Servings: 1 | Total time: 6 min

Calories: 144 Kcal, | Fat: 14g | Protein: 14g | Carbohydrates: 4g

Ingredients

o   Unsweetened almond milk 1/2 cup

o   Heavy whipping cream 2 tbsp

o   Cocoa powder 1 tbsp

o   Salted caramel collagen 1 to 2 tbsp

o   Liquid sweetener

o   Whipped cream

o   Caramel sauce

Steps of preparation

o   Combine almond or the hemp milk and heavy cream in a pan over medium heat. Get it to a boil.

o   In a mixer, incorporate the chocolate powder and the collagen. Put in the hot milk and mix until the milk is frothy.

o   Top with thinly sweetened ice cream and a caramel sauce to top it off!

12. Ketogenic brownie bark

Servings: 12　| Total time: 45 min

Calories: 98 Kcal, | Fat: 8.3g | Protein: 2.4g | Carbohydrates: 4.3g

Ingredients

o　Almond flour 1/2 cup

o　Baking powder 1/2 tsp

o　Salt 1/4 tsp

o　Room temperature 2 leg whites

o　Swerve sweetener 1/2 cup

o　Cocoa powder 3 tbsp

o　Instant coffee 1 tsp

o　Butter melted 1/4 cup

o　Heavy whipping cream 1 tbsp

o　Vanilla 1/2 tsp

o　Chocolate chips 1/3 cups

Steps of Preparation

o　Start by preheating the oven to 325F and place parchment paper on a baking sheet. Lubricate the parchment paper with oil.

o　In a small cup, mix together the flour, baking powder and the salt.

o　Mix the egg whites in a large bowl until it becomes foggy. Mix in the sweetener, chocolate powder and some instant coffee until it becomes smooth and then mix in the melted butter, cream and the vanilla. Mix in a mixture with almond flour until it is well mixed.

o　Now spread the batter on the lubricated parchment in a square of around 12 by 12 inches. Sprinkle some chocolate chips.

o　Now bake for 18 minutes, until it is puffed and all set. Remove from the oven, turn the oven off and let it cool for 15 minutes.

o　Using a sharp knife, cut through 2-inch squares, but do not detach. Return to a warm oven for about 5 to 10 minutes and toast lightly.

o　Remove, let it cool fully, then divide into squares.

13. Ketogenic Homemade Nutella

Servings: 6 | Total time: 20 min

Calories: 158 Kcal, |Fat: 18.3g |Protein: 3.3g | Carbohydrates: 18 g

Ingredients

o   Hazelnuts toasted 3/4 cup

o   Coconut oil 2 to 3 tbsp

o   Cocoa powder 2 tbsp

o   Powdered swerve sweetener 2 tbsp

o   Vanilla extract 1/2 tsp

o   Pinch salt

Steps of Preparation

o   Grind hazelnuts in a processor until finely ground and starts to clump together.

o   Now add two tablespoons oil and keep on grinding until the nuts become smooth out. Add remaining of the ingredients and then blend until well mixed. in case of thick mixture, add one more tablespoon oil.

14. Ketogenic snickerdoodle truffles

Servings: 24 truffles yield | Total time: 20 min

Calories: 150 Kcal, |Fat: 14g |Protein: 3g | Carbohydrates: 13 g

Ingredients

o   Almond flour 2 cups

o   Swerve 1/2 cup

o   Cream of tartar 1 tsp

o   Ground cinnamon 1 tsp

o   Salt 1/4 tsp

o   Butter 6 tbsp

o   Vanilla extract 1 tsp

o   Swerve 3 tbsp

o   Ground cinnamon 1 tsp

Steps of preparation

o   In a large bowl, mix together the Swerve, the cream of tartar, the almond flour, cinnamon, and the salt. Now stir in melted butter and some vanilla extract till the dough is combined. Add a tablespoon of water in case of hard dough and stir together.

o   Now scoop dough with rounded tablespoon and then squeeze in the palm and hold together, now roll into a ball. Transfer on a waxed paper which is lined on a cookie sheet, and then repeat.

o   In a small bowl, mix together the cinnamon and the Swerve. Now roll the truffles in this coating.

o   Serve.

15. Chocolate chip keto cookies

Servings: 20 | Total time: 30 min

Calories: 238 kcal | Proteins: 4.3 g | Carbohydrates: 8.18 g | Fat:21.5 g

Ingredients

o   Almond flour 1 1/4 cups

o   Unsweetened coconut 3/4 cups

o   Baking powder 1 tsp

o   Salt 1/2 tsp

o   Butter softened 1/2 cup

o   Swerve sweetener 1/2 cup

o   Yacon syrup or molasses 2 tsp

o   Vanilla extract 1/2 tsp

o   Egg 1 large

o   Chocolate chips sugar-free 1 cup

Steps of preparation

o   Start by preheating the oven to a temperature of 325F and then line a baking sheet with the parchment paper.

o   In a small bowl, mix together some almond flour, baking powder, salt and coconut.

o   In a big bowl, add cream butter and the Swerve Sweetener along with molasses. Add in vanilla and egg, beat until well mixed. Now beat in some flour mixture till dough is well mixed completely.

o Mix in some chocolate chips.

o Now shape the dough into small balls and then place them 2 inches apart on the lined baking sheet. Press the ball to a 1/4 inch of thickness.

o Now bake 12 to 15 minutes, till just starts to brown.

o Let cool completely on the pan after removing from oven.

o Serve.

16. Keto Fat Bomb with jam and Peanut butter

Servings: 12 | Total time: 45 min

Calories: 223 kcal | Proteins: 3.8 g | Carbohydrates: 4.5 g | Fat:21.5 g

Ingredients

o Raspberries 3/4 cup

o Water 1/4 cup

o powdered Swerve Sweetener 6 to 8 tbsp

o grass-fed gelatin 1 tsp

o creamy peanut butter 3/4 cup

o coconut oil 3/4 cup

Steps of preparation

o Fill a muffin tin with 12 liners of parchment paper.

o Mix the raspberries and water in a small saucepan. Bring it to a boil and lower the heat and simmer for 5 minutes. Now mash the berries with your fork.

o Mix in 2 to 4 tbsp of powdered sweetener, based on how sweet you want. Mix in the peanut butter and gelatin and let it cool.

o Mix peanut butter and the coconut oil in a microwave safe jar. Cook on maximum for 30 to 60 seconds, once it has melted. Whisk the powdered sweetener in 2 to 4 tbsp, depending about how sweet you want it.

o Partition half of peanut butter mixture into 12 cups and put in the freezer for around 15 minutes. Divide the mixture of raspberry between the cups then top with the remaining mixture of peanut butter.

o Chill in refrigerator until becomes solid.

17. Classic Blueberry Scones

Servings: 12 | Total time: 40 min

Calories: 223 kcal | Proteins: 5.5 g | Carbohydrates: 7.21 g | Fat:12 g

Ingredients

o   <u>Almond flour</u> 2 cups

o   <u>swerve sweetener</u> 1/3 cup

o   <u>coconut flour</u> 1/4 cup

o   Baking powder 1 tbsp

o   Tsp salt 1/4

o   Eggs 2 large

o   Heavy whipping cream 1/4 cup

o   <u>Vanilla extract</u> 1/2 tsp

o   Fresh blueberries 3/4 cup

Steps of Preparation

o   Preheat the oven to 325F and cover a big baking sheet with a silicone lining or a parchment paper.

o   In a big bowl, mix together the rice, coconut flour, the baking powder, sweetener, and salt.

o   Mix in the eggs, whipped cream and vanilla and combine until the dough starts to combine. Include the blueberries.

o   Assemble the dough together and now place on the prepared baking sheet. Put in a rugged rectangle measuring 10 x 8 inches.

o   Using a sharp, broad knife to break into six squares. Then split each of these squares laterally into the two triangles. Gently raise the scones and then scatter them across the tray.

o   Bake for almost 25 minutes until becomes golden brown. Remove it and leave it cool.

o   Serve.

18. Chocolate coconut cups

Servings: 20 | Total time: 20 min

Calories: 223 kcal | Proteins: 5.5 g | Carbohydrates: 7.21 g | Fat:12 g

Ingredients

o Coconut butter 1/2 cup

o Kelapo coconut oil 1/2 cup

o Unsweetened coconut 1/2 cup

o Powdered swerve sweetener 3 tbsp

o Ounces cocoa butter 1 & 1/2

o Unsweetened chocolate 1 ounce

o Powdered swerve sweetener 1/4 cup

o Cocoa powder 1/4 cup

o Vanilla extract 1/4 tsp

Steps of preparation

o For candies, cover a mini muffin tray with a 20 mini paper lining.

o Mix coconut butter and the coconut oil in a small saucepan over low flame. Stir until melted and creamy, then mix in the shredded coconut and the sweetener until merged.

o Divide the mixture between the prepared muffin cups and then freeze until solid, for around 30 minutes.

o For chocolate coating, mix cocoa butter and the unsweetened chocolate in a bowl placed on a pan of simmering water. Stir until it has melted.

o Mix in the sifted powdered sweetener and now stir in cocoa powder until smooth.

o Now remove from the heat and whisk in the extract of vanilla.

o Put chocolate topping over the coconut candies and then let it cook for around 15 minutes.

o Candies can be kept on your kitchen countertop for up to one week.

19. Roll biscotti

Servings: 15 | Total time: 1 hr. 20 min

Calories: 123 kcal | Proteins: 4 g | Carbohydrates: 4 g | Fat:12 g

Ingredients

o Swerve Sweetener 2 tbsp

o Ground cinnamon 1 tsp

o Almond flour Honeyville 2 cups

o   Swerve Sweetener 1/3 cup

o   Baking powder 1 tsp

o   Xanthan gum 1/2 tsp

o   Salt 1/4 tsp

o   Melted butter 1/4 cup

o   Egg 1 large

o   Vanilla extract 1 tsp

o   Swerve Sweetener 1/4 cup

o   Heavy cream 2 tbsp

o   Vanilla 1/2 tsp

Steps of preparation

o   In a small bowl, combine the sweetener and the cinnamon for filling. Set it apart.

o   Preheat the oven to a temperature of 325F, cover the baking sheet with the parchment paper.

o   In a big bowl, whisk together the starch, baking powder, the xanthan gum, sweetener, and salt. Stir in 1/4 cup of butter, the egg and the vanilla extract before the dough fits together.

o   Turn the dough onto the lined baking sheet and then half it in two. Shape each half into a rectangular shape of around 10 by 4 inches. Making sure the scale and form of both halves are identical.

o   Sprinkle with around 2/3 of cinnamon filling. Cover with one of the other parts of the dough, close the seams and then smooth the cover.

o   Bake for almost 25 minutes or until gently browned and solid to the touch. Transfer from the oven and spray the remaining melted butter on it, then dust with the leftover cinnamon mixture. Allow it to cool for about 30 minutes and reduce the temperature to 250F.

o   Cut log into around 15 slices with sharp knife.

o   Place the slices back on the cut-side in the baking sheet and bake for another 15 minutes, then turn over and bake for the next 15 minutes. Turn the oven off and let it stay within until it's cold.

20. Garahm crackers
Servings: 10 | Total time: 1 hr. 5 min

Calories: 156 kcal | Proteins: 5 g | Carbohydrates: 6 g | Fat:13 g

Ingredients

o   Almond flour 2 cups

o   Swerve brown 1/3 cup

o   Cinnamon 2 tsp

o   Baking powder 1 tsp

o   A pinch of salt

o   Egg 1 large

o   Butter melted 2 tbsp

o   Vanilla extract 1 tsp

Steps of preparation

o   Preheat the oven to 300F for crackers.

o   In a big cup, stir together flour, cinnamon, baking powder, sweetener, and salt. Stir in egg, melted butter, molasses and vanilla extract before the dough falls together.

o   Transform the dough into a wide sheet of parchment paper and pat into a rough rectangle. Cover with a sheet of parchment. Print out the dough to around 1/8-inch thickness as uniformly as possible.

o   Cut the top of the parchment and now use a sharp knife to rank around 2x2 inches in squares. Move the whole piece of parchment to the baking sheet.

o   Bake for 20 to 30 minutes, until brown and strong. Remove the crackers and let them cool for 30 minutes, then split up along the score. Return to the warm oven if it's so far cooled off, turn it on and adjust the temperature to no higher than 200F). Let it sit for yet another 30 minutes, then cool absolutely.

Conclusion

This book explained keto diet in detail, which is a high-fat, low-carbohydrate diet similar to Atkins & low-carb diets. It involves substantially reducing the consumption of carbohydrates and replacing them with fat. After reading this book, you will several unique concerns and subjects that relate mainly or exclusively to women over 50 on keto diet.   There are some key takeaways for women above 50 on keto Diet and the problems one has to be aware of. After reading this book, you will learn some easy, rapid and simple recipes for women above 50. These include the breakfast, lunch and the dinner keto-based recipes, which are low in carbohydrates. This book also presented some delicious snacks and smoothies too. Some exercise and gym friendly recipes are also presented.

The 15-Day Keto Fasting Cookbook

A Sophisticated Mix of Low-Carb Recipes to Activate Ketosis and Autophagy for Life-Long Intermittent Fasting

By

Stacey Bell

Table of Contents

Introduction

Given the multiple kinds of diets you have probably read about in your life, you are likely to have a few fresh ones. Perhaps one amongst them may be the Ketogenic Diet, commonly known as the Keto Diet, which is a low-carbohydrate, high-fat regimen.

The idea behind the high-fat, low-carbohydrate ratio is that instead of carbs, the body would depend on fats for nutrition, and hence the body would become leaner as a consequence of getting less fat contained throughout the body.

Ideally, the Keto Diet would encourage the body to achieve ketosis or a metabolic condition where the carbs are ketones, which are fats that are burned for energy rather than glucose. Many who embrace the Keto Diet often eat only the correct amount of protein on a regular basis that the body requires. The Keto Diet does not rely on measuring calories, compared to any of the other diets that occur. Instead, the emphasis is on the food's fat, proteins and carbohydrates make-up, as well as the weight of the servings.

But what contributed to the Keto Diet being created?

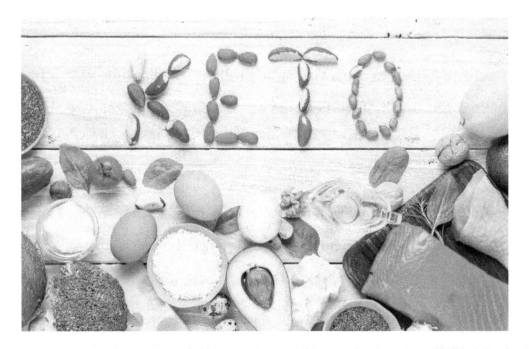

In hopes of discovering a cure for seizures, a Mayo Clinic physician by the name of Russell Wilder invented the Ketogenic Diet back in 1924. Since going on this diet, many people who have epilepsy and other disorders have reported a substantial reduction in their symptoms. This procedure goes back to Ancient Greece when physicians would change the diets of their patients and even make them rapidly push their bodies into hunger mode.

The Ketogenic Diet is a much better way for the body to reach the fasting mode without completely depriving the body of food. However, to this day, no one understands precisely why the Ketogenic Diet is so effective in treating those who have epilepsy, autism, and other identified diseases.

The high-fat, low-carbohydrate combination might be a normal meal for those on the Ketogenic Diet, which would include a balanced portion of some fruit or a protein-rich vegetable, protein such as chicken and a high-fat portion that may be butter. The high-fat portion of this diet typically comes from the food-making ingredients; this may involve heavy cream, butter, or buttermilk, and creamy dressings such as ranch could also be mixed.

Unfortunately, with its potential for instantaneous results, this natural approach to healing had to give way to the new advancement of medicinal research.

Happily, again and perhaps for really good purposes, the ketogenic diet has made its way back into the spotlight!

You see, the cornerstone of the diet is to effectively stimulate the fat-burning processes of your own body to feel what the body wants for energy during the day. This implies that all the fat you consume and the accumulated fat in your body have both been fuel reserves that can be taped over by your body! No wonder that except among some persistent, hard to lose fat regions, this plan also helps you with weight reduction. It may be one of the explanations why you selected this eBook and looked into the ketogenic process, or you might have learned stories from your social group on how the keto diet really normalizes blood glucose levels and optimizes the cholesterol measurements and you are fascinated. Only by adopting this plan alone, how about the news of type 2 diabetes getting cured as well as stories of some diseases being prevented or tumors shrinking thanks to the beneficial impact of the keto diet? Even as a result of the diet, we do overlook the risk of heart disease!

All the above-mentioned advantages derive primarily from a single major mechanism in the ketogenic diet. The name of the game is ketosis.

In this very book, all information about the keto diet and intermittent fasting is provided and lets you know how it's helpful for quick and healthy weight loss.

Chapter 1- Ketogenic Diet and Ketosis

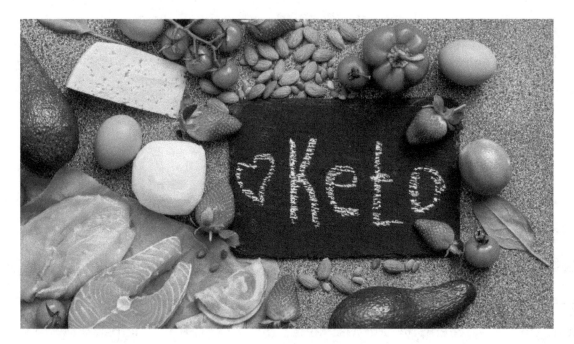

You may be on a ketogenic diet or are contemplating it.

If you desire to kickstart with ketosis, then your ticket is for intermittent fasting.

Truth be known, it can be daunting to follow a ketogenic diet, mainly because there are too many things that you cannot consume. But be assured the truth-ketosis is spiritual.

Fortunately, whether you don't want to eat a ketogenic diet, you will easily get a route to ketosis.

When the body burns up ketones and fat for food instead of glucose, ketosis happens.

In two cases, that happens:

1. there is no food coming (fasting) or

2. little or no carbohydrates come through (ketogenic dieting).

It regularly makes ketones in the process when your system is in the fat-burning phase; hence, you are in ketosis.

For the body to be in the process of ketosis is perfectly natural, and it was definitely a popular occurrence for humans across history that had intermittent accessibility to food and fasting times in between. For those following a Western diet, though, the physiological condition of ketosis is very unusual since we are all feeding. You basically get negligible ketones in your blood while you're consuming something else than a ketogenic diet. But it's very rare for our generation of people to be in a condition of ketosis unless you seek one out purposefully.

Post 8 hours of fasting, as you wake up, ketone levels are only starting to raise. Ketone output will speed up to provide more of the energy you need if you prolong your fast until noon, and your body will finally be in the renowned fat-burning condition of ketosis. If you want to manage to burn body fat at a high pace by keeping to your fast for 16 hours or a day or a few days, and not by consuming anything ketogenic, you need to live in ketosis!

A lot of focus is given to reaching ketosis through ketogenic diets, but if you consume keto foods, where do you suppose any of the ketones come from? And not the fat on the thighs and hips. Fasting for ketosis means that only the body fat comes from the ketones that feed the brain, thereby getting rid of it.

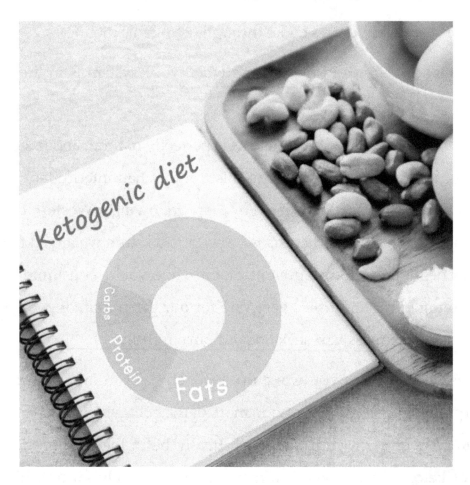

Ketosis is a condition in which the body creates compounds that are formed by the liver, labeled ketones. Crafted to supply organs and cells with nutrition, it may substitute sugar as an additional source of food. We get much of our energy from glucose in our conventional diet, rich in carbs which are processed from the carbohydrates that we consume throughout meals. Glucose is a fast energy supply, where insulin is needed as a kind of intermediary that tells the cells to open up and enables the flow of glucose so that it can be used as a mitochondrial fuel, better known as the fuel factories in our cells. The further sugars we eat, the more glucose is found in our blood, which suggests that the pancreas has to generate more insulin to promote the extraction of energy from usable blood sugar. In an organism where the metabolism is still natural, the cells readily embrace the insulin released by the pancreas, which then contributes to the effective use of blood glucose as energy. The concern is that our cells will actually become desensitized to insulin, contributing to a condition in which the pancreas is required to inject more and more insulin into the bloodstream only to clear the blood sugar levels and normalize them.

Insulin de-sensitivity or insulin tolerance is primarily induced by the constant enhanced presence of blood glucose and is typically caused by the intake of foods high in carbon. Picture of the cells of the body like a security guard at a bar, where you need to pay a charge to enter the club. Here, you play a glucose function, and the cost paid to join the club is insulin. If the club intensity is in accordance with the standard, the security officer doesn't really notice something odd and does not increase the admission fee needed. However, if you wake up clamoring to be allowed in just about every night, the bouncer understands the dire need and jacks up the insulin charge periodically in order to let glucose in. Gradually, at such a stage that the source of insulin, which in this situation is the pancreas, no longer generates any, the admission fee grows greater and greater. This is when the situation is diagnosed with type 2 diabetes, and the normal solution will include drugs or insulin injections for a lifetime. In the existence of glucose in the body system lies the crux of the matter here. Our blood sugar levels are raised every time we take in a carb-rich meal, which is not complicated in this day and age of fast food and sugary snacks, and insulin is enabled for the conversion into energy as well as the storage of the wasted waste into fat cells. This is where the normal furor begins, with condemnations pouring in as the cause of numerous ailments and dreaded weight gain with both glucose and insulin. It wouldn't be wrong if it claimed that insulin and glucose, as certain books have made them out to be, are most certainly not the source of all bad. To refer to our present diet as the leading cause of metabolic disorders and obesity plaguing the greater part of the developing world will be much more specific.

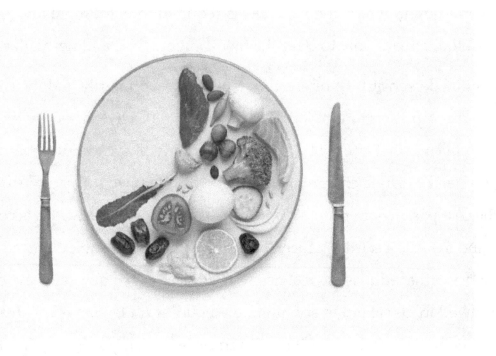

Link the ketogenic diet, which is where the shift toward the positive will be seen.

The keto diet, with a focus on being intentionally low carb, is a fat-based diet. This strategy is intended to decrease our consumption of sugar and starchy foods that are too easily affordable. Just a pleasant fact: in the old days, sugar was actually used as a preservative, and it's no accident that a number of the packaged goods we have now involve massive quantities of sugar so that it makes for longer shelf life. The hedonic appetite reaction in the brain has often been found to cause foods rich in sugar, ultimately allowing you to feed for the sake of gratification rather than actual hunger. Studies also found that sugar therapies are linked to the regions of the brain that are often responsible for opioid use and gambling. You know now that it appears like you can't resist tossing those caramelized sweets into the mouth.

So, we cut back on sugars, and this is where the fat comes in to offset the calories required to help the body. You will be looking at taking seventy-five percent of the daily calorie as fats on the regular ketogenic diet, approximately twenty percent as protein and the remaining five percent in the form of carbohydrates. We are doing it because, as we know, we want our key source of fuel to be fat. We will cause the body to induce ketosis only with the mixture of cutting down carbohydrates and growing our fat intake. We either do so with a diet that makes long-term, safe use, or we actually starve through ketosis. Yeah, sure, you heard it correctly; ketosis is the normal mechanism of the body that creates a shield against the lean periods where there is a lack of food.

Chapter 2- Intermittent fasting and the ketogenic diet

In recent years, this has also been bandied about a lot, with some seeking to shed a misleading light on the keto diet by associating it with thirst.

To make it simpler, when our bodies feel that we do not have adequate glucose in the bloodstream, the ketosis mechanism is initiated. In order to ensure the continuous availability of nutrition for our cells and tissues, it then switches to our fat reserves to transform them into ketones via the liver. It does not mean that you are necessarily killing yourself on the keto diet! Any time someone says that, he got a little worked up.

How will a person who eats 1,800 to 2,000 calories on a regular basis, which is what you're going to get on the meal plan, starve effectively?

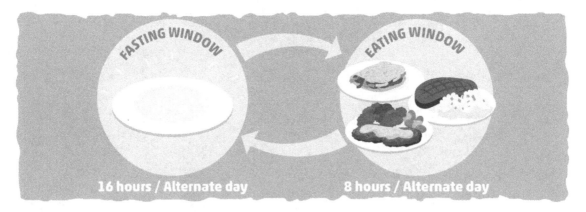

To be fair, during the hunter-gatherer days of our human past, ketosis comes in very handy. This was a time where agriculture wasn't that common, and what you searched or found relied on the food you consumed. This produced a scenario where there could be no calories for days at a time, so our bodies sent insulin to ferry it through our organs as glucose made its way through the environment, as well as hoarding the leftover glucose into fat cells for potential usage.

The body then reached the condition of ketosis by using the accumulated fats to provide nutrition during the lean periods when there was really little food to be found.

Our hunger hormones, like ghrelin, decrease their development during this stage, and the hormones that regulate satiety, like leptin, see their levels increased. All this is how our bodies want to make the most of it to make it easier for us to feel as comfortable as possible if nutritional supplies are scarce.

Today, quick forward to modern days, where food is practically only one or two streets away, or maybe just a car ride away, and we're not going to experience food scarcity like our predecessors in the Paleolithic. However, our bodies also retain the processes and pathways that have enabled them to function. That is the main explanation why we reduce carbohydrates and raise our regular fat consumption on the keto diet.

The condition of ketosis is triggered when we do so, and we get to reap all the biochemical advantages that the diet confers.

The fat we consume often goes into replenishing the body's fat reserves, which is why it won't be wrong to claim again when on the ketogenic diet, one should not starve!

How the Intermitting Fasting Works

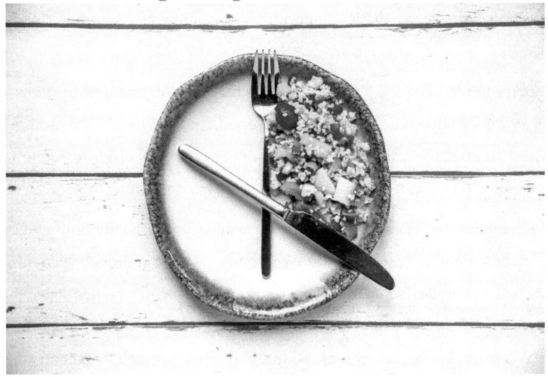

From the context of weight reduction, intermittent fasting operates by finding it more challenging to overeat during the day. A basic guideline such as "skip breakfast" or "eat only between 5 pm and 8 pm" will help keep you from reaching for sweets or consuming calorie-dense drinks that lead to weight gain during the day.

You'll also find it impossible to overeat, even though you work up a ferocious appetite when fasting. In fact, intermittent fasting appears to decrease the intake of daily energy and encourage fat loss.

This ensures that as long as you adhere to a shorter feeding time or a fixed number of meals, you can be willing to consume as much as you like and meet your objectives.

Your body may need to adapt itself to this new eating pattern when you first attempt intermittent fasting. Hunger pangs and strong cravings may strike you hard at first, but they will soon recede when your cells feast on accumulated fat and ketones.

Insulin removal, ketone synthesis and autophagy are the main pathways behind your ability to quickly lose weight and boost your health in the process. Our insulin levels drop incrementally as we accumulate time in a fasting condition. This facilitates the liberation of fat from our fat cells and activates the mechanism known as ketogenesis that generates ketones.

You'll reach a deeper state of ketosis as you continue your easy, become more successful at burning fat, and speed up the self-cleaning mechanism known as autophagy.

Benefits of Intermitting Fasting

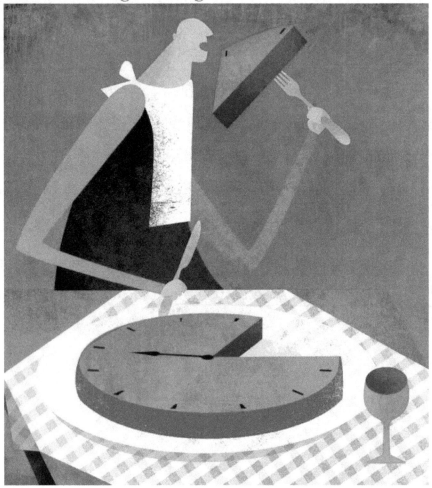

1. Enhanced regulation of blood sugar and resistance to insulin

This will also help boost blood sugar levels and improve one's cells' insulin response by allowing the body an occasional break from calorie intake. One research study showed that for six meals a day, intermittent fasting could also be a healthier option than having the same calorie deficit.

The two dietary strategies can function synergistically to boost blood sugar regulation when paired with the keto diet, which has also been shown to assist with insulin tolerance and type 2 diabetes. More study on the results of using them in tandem, however, is needed.

2. Psychic Clarity

Your brain will essentially operate on ketones, which are extracted through fat dissolution in the liver until the body is keto-adapted.

Fat is thought to be one of the body's most energy-efficient resources to work on, and your mind is a major energy user.

When you do not regularly refill on grains and fruits, most high-carb supporters fight for the malnutrition your body endures. They expect you to take a granola bar and an apple around you everywhere you go, but the advantage of Keto is that you don't.

And if the body is full of glycogen (which is more definitely if you are in ketosis), the excess of fat from the meals you consume and shop you have will depend on it. That ensures that your brain powerhouse will operate at maximum capacity all the time. Less emotional fogginess and more attention.

You can begin to lose fat automatically when you get used to dieting. In other terms, feed only when you are starving. Don't arrange the fasting; let it arise spontaneously.

3. Fitness

People still claim that if you don't use the benefit of pre-and post-exercise meals while you work out, you're going to lose muscle.

This is not inherently real, and when you're adapted to ketosis, it is much less so.

In the long run, fasting while practicing can contribute to a variety of advantages, including:

1. **Greater mutation adaptations** - Studies indicate that when you work out in a fasting condition, your training efficiency will improve in the long run.

2. **Enhanced muscle synthesis**- Experiments indicate that when you exercise in a fasting condition and use sufficient nutrient consumption, muscle gains are improved.

3. **Increased reaction to post-workout meals**-Studies suggests that the accelerated ingestion of nutrients after a short exercise will contribute to better outcomes.

Mechanism Behind the Benefits

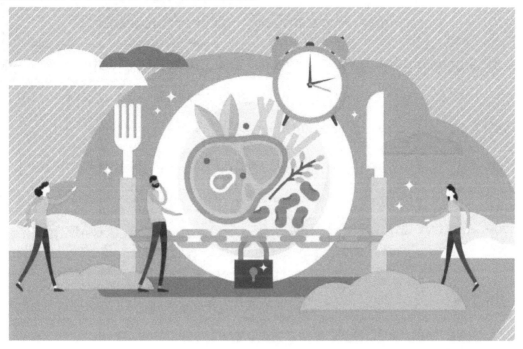

Intermittent fasting is so effective that it can be used to reduce calories, trigger ketosis, and enable the mechanisms of autophagy induced by protein restriction and hunger.

This is what happens to our cells as we consume three or more meals a day, which meets our normal calorie requirements fully. Your cells will also be backed up with non-essential proteins and poisonous chemicals, sometimes after consuming the healthiest diets, but what can you do?

You soon, not from cooking, but from being consumed by other commitments, to ensure you clean your real bedroom. You need to fast with food to ensure sure the cells will clean themselves.

Not only can this fasting phase trigger this cleanup for your cells, but it will increase the output of your ketones and facilitate fat burning as well. Simply stated, by incorporating intermittent fasting into the keto diet, coupled with the consequences of autophagy, you can enjoy the advantages of Keto more easily.

In addition, you will raise ketone amounts, lose more fat, and improve autophagy more than you can with intermittent fasting alone if you begin to implement intermittent fasting and exercise together.

Overall, the evidence for intermittent fasting shows that it will be a perfect complement to the keto lifestyle for certain persons, whether you include activity or not. Before you start, though, it is important to be acquainted with the unpleasant signs that can occur.

Chapter 3- How autophagy and ketosis are synergic?

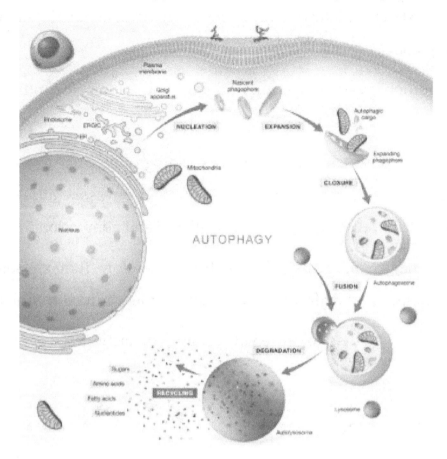

In order to reconstruct healthy, healthier cells, autophagy is the body's method of wiping out dead cells.

Auto" implies self, and "phagy" implies eating." So, 'self-eating' is the literal sense of autophagy.

That is often referred to as "self-devouring." Although it might seem like something you would wish to occur to your body, your ultimate wellbeing is actually advantageous.

It is since autophagy is an evolved method of self-preservation by which the organism can extract and regenerate sections of dysfunctional cells for cellular repair and hygiene.

The aim of autophagy is to eliminate debris and return to optimum smooth operation through self-regulation.

Around the same moment, it's recycling and washing, almost like touching the body on a reset button. Plus, as a reaction to different stressors and contaminants accumulated in our bodies, it encourages resilience and adaptation.

Note that autophagy simply means "self-eating." Therefore, it makes sense that it is understood that intermittent fasting and ketogenic diets induce autophagy.

The most successful method to cause autophagy is by fasting.

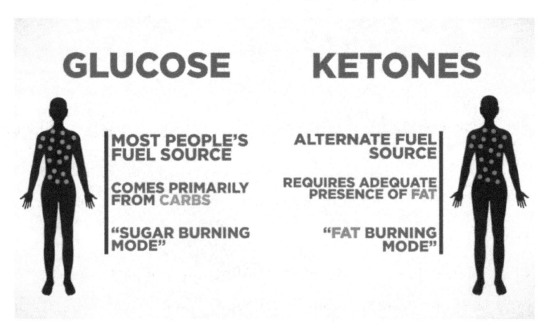

Ketosis, a high-fat and low-carb diet, offers the same advantages to eating without fasting, such as a shortcut that causes the same advantageous biochemical adjustments. It allows the body a break to concentrate on its own wellbeing and repair by not stressing the body with an external load.

You receive about 75 percent of the recommended daily calories from fat in the keto diet and 5 to 10 percent of your calories from carbohydrates.

This alteration in calorie sources allows the biochemical processes in the body to change. Instead of the glucose that is extracted from carbohydrates, it would start using fat for food.

In reaction to this ban, the body will begin to start creating ketone bodies that have several protective effects. Khorana says studies show that ketosis, which has neuroprotective functions, may also cause starvation-induced autophagy.

In all diets, low glucose levels exist and are related to low insulin and high levels of glucagon. And the degree of glucagon is the one that initiates autophagy.

It brings the constructive stress that wakes up the survival repair mode when the body is low on sugar by fasting or ketosis.

Exercise is one non-diet region that can also play a part in causing autophagy. Physical activity can, according to one animal research, cause autophagy in organs that are part of the processes of metabolic control.

Chapter 4- Keto Diet and weight loss

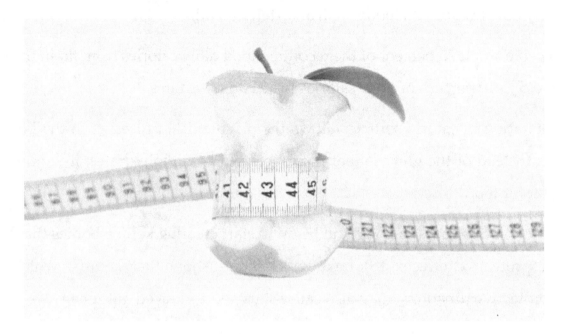

When we start on a ketogenic diet, one of the first items we still lose is most certainly water weight. As adipose fats, the body stores glucose, although there is a limited supply of glucose that is processed as glycogen, composed mainly of water. Glycogen is intended to provide rapid bursting capacity, the kind we use when we run or raise weights. The body switches to glycogen as the first source of energy supply as we cut carbohydrates, which is why water weight is lost in the initial phases. This initial blast of weight reduction may be a morale booster for everyone, and for people who conform to the keto diet, it is a positive signpost for what is to come. Water weight is readily lost and gained, as a side note. This suggests that even those who first see certain outcomes in the keto diet and then wish to get off the track for some reason, as carbohydrates become the daily calorie mainstay, the odds are their weight would swell back up.

For the rest that conforms to the ketogenic diet, what comes next will be the fat burning process of the body that is responsible for the impressive effects of weight loss shown by many. The underlying principle is also the same in that adipose fats are still activated by the organs and cells of the body as energy sources, contributing to a normal state of depletion of fat and thus accompanying reducing weight.

The burning of fat is not the sole explanation that the keto diet demonstrates weight reduction.

Hunger reduction and improvement of pleasure during meals are also explanations that people are better able to lose weight whilst on a diet. One of the long-standing ideals of weight management has always been the adage of drinking less and doing more. The entire premise is to establish a calorie shortage in such a way that the body is forced to depend on its stored energy reserves to make up for the requisite expenditure. That seems quick and straightforward on paper, but it may be as challenging as scaling Mount Everest for someone who has been through scenarios where you have had to deliberately curtail your food on a hungry stomach!

Through the ketogenic diet, thanks to the modification of the hormones that regulate sensations of appetite and fullness, you realize that you will have normal hunger suppression. In addition, the food we usually eat while on a diet often assists with weight reduction. It is understood that fats and protein are more relaxing and rewarding than sugary carbs. We do two items almost concurrently as we turn to a high-fat diet when cutting back on the carbohydrates. Only because we feel like it, not because we are very hungry, easing back on carbohydrates, particularly the sugar stuff, reduces the urge to consume. Charging high the consumption of fat often causes the satiety impact even easier and helps you to feel complete. This is part of so many keto dieters claim that without having the smallest pinch of hunger, they will go for two and a half or even two meals a day.

We account for a regular caloric consumption that varies from 1,800 to 2,000 calories on our keto meal schedule, but we do not even use calorie limits to minimize weight. The truth is that those tiny and harmless-looking snacks that fill the period between dinners will not appear much in your life when you feel fullness and enjoyment from your meals! Think about it: the usual go-to sweets, donuts, candy, and cookies, are left out purely, so you are less inclined to give in to hedonistic appetite induced mainly by the same sugar treats in reducing extra calories which would have otherwise been converted to adipose fat tissue, that goes a very long way.

To sum up, without the usual calorie limit in most weight reduction diets, the ketogenic diet provides for meals. It also offers a supporting hand in the production of symptoms of hunger suppression such that you do not have to struggle with those treacherous hunger pangs! The lack of carb munchies is also present, which may theoretically disrupt any diet. With as minimal disturbance to our everyday life as possible, this helps one to experience normal weight loss. There is no need to deploy calorie counters, no need for a problematic six to eight meals a day, and certainly no strange or amusing workout exercises required. If you pair it with the satisfying high-fat keto meals, you enter a scenario where hunger could indeed become an outsider.

As another good spin-off, having to re-learn what real hunger feels like still arrives. We get incidents of hunger on a carb-rich diet, and our blood sugar levels appear to fluctuate dramatically as our cells become increasingly desensitized by insulin. The propensity to feed on impulse is often enhanced by sugar, which can really ruin any diet! We will also have to wake up and take care anytime we feel those hunger pangs when we cut back on carbohydrates and ratchet up on the fats, so that will be proper signs that the body needs extra energy.

Chapter 5- Benefits of Ketogenic Diet

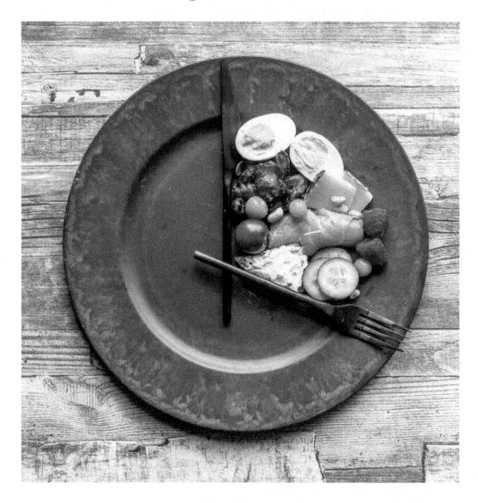

All in all, the straightforward method to the keto diet has inspired individuals to engage with it, resulting in many variants of the keto diet that are available. The keto diet method has been one of the most attempted regimes, and in the last few years, it has grown tremendously in prominence.

Although the key advantage of Keto is successful weight loss, metabolic boosting and hunger control, such advantages include the following-

1. Acne may be decreased by the keto diet since glucose restriction can tip the dynamics of bacteria in the intestine that influences the face.

2. It is known to deter and cure some cancers and, in addition to radiation and chemotherapy, is seen as a supportive medication since it allows cancer cells to undergo additional oxidative stress, allowing them to die.

3. This diet provides your body with a better and healthy source of energy and thus will make you feel more energetic throughout the day.

4. A reduction in cholesterol is caused by keto diets, and the presence of healthy cholesterol is improved.

5. The brain and nerve cells are reinforced and preserved. In addition, it is understood to manage diseases such as Alzheimer's, Parkinson's etc.

6. Many types of research have shown that the keto diet helps to lower down the low-density lipoproteins or the bad cholesterol over time and have been shown to eliminate diseases such as type 2 diabetes.

7. It aids in losing weight as the body burns down the fat as the prior energy source, and one will primarily be using the fat stored in the body as an energy source while in a fasting mode.

8. A Keto diet has been shown to improve cholesterol levels and triglyceride levels most associated with arterial buildup.

9. Known for managing epilepsy-like disorders, Ovarian polycystic disease, etc.

10. The ketogenic diet promises many keto advantages, but a true effort is to initiate the keto diet. It is a restrictive diet that seeks to reduce one's carb consumption to about 50 grams a day, so visiting a dietician to work out and modify the diet according to one's needs is advantageous.

Chapter 6- The 15-day Meal Plan with Low-Carb Recipes that fit the Intermittent Fasting Diet

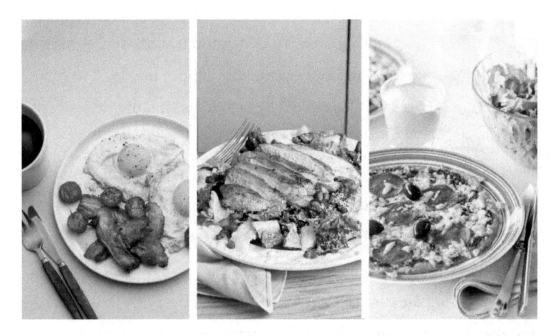

Eating Keto involves limiting the net carb consumption such that energy and ketones are generated by your body metabolizing fat. For many, this means reducing net carbs to 20 grams a day.

The keto diet could be perfect for you if you are trying to optimize advantages such as curing type 2 diabetes or if you want to lose the extra kilos

A more balanced low-carb diet could be a safer option for you if you want more carbohydrates in your diet and if you don't have type 2 diabetes or have a lot of weight to lose. It may be better to adopt mild low carb, but it may also be less successful than Keto, suggesting you may get more modest outcomes.

Day 1

Breakfast- Scrambled eggs

Lunch-Bacon and Zucchini Noodles Salad

Dinner- Spinach Soup

Day 2

Breakfast- Keto Frittata

Lunch-Keto Roasted Pepper and Cauliflower

Dinner-Buffalo Blue Cheese Chicken Wedges

Day 3

Breakfast- Breakfast Bowl

Lunch-Lunch Tacos

Dinner-Lemon Dill Trout

Day 4

Breakfast- Poached Eggs

Lunch-Simple Pizza Rolls

Dinner-Special Fish Pie

Day 5

Breakfast- Bright Morning Smoothie

Lunch-Lunch Stuffed Peppers

Dinner-Cauliflower Bread Garlic Sticks

Day 6

Breakfast-Pumpkin Muffins

Lunch-Lunch Stuffed Peppers

Dinner- Buffalo Blue Cheese Chicken Wedges

Day 7

Breakfast- Keto Breakfast Mix

Lunch-Lunch Caesar Salad

Dinner-Sage N Orange Breast of Duck

Day 8

Breakfast-Pumpkin Pie Spiced Latte

Lunch-Keto Roasted Pepper and Cauliflower

Dinner- Salmon with Caper Sauce

Day 9

Breakfast- Strawberry Protein Smoothie

Lunch-Keto Slow Cooker Buffalo Chicken Soup

Dinner-Cauliflower Bread Garlic Sticks

Day 10

Breakfast-Delicious Eggs and Sausages

Lunch-Special Lunch Burgers

Dinner-Tossed Brussel Sprout Salad

Day 11

Breakfast-Bright Morning Smoothie

Lunch-Keto Lunch Jambalaya

Dinner- Spinach Soup

Day 12

Breakfast-Keto Frittata

Lunch-Lunch Tacos

Dinner-Special Fish Pie

Day 13

Breakfast-Feta and Asparagus Delight

Lunch-Keta Chicken Enchilada Soup

Dinner-Bok Choy Stir Fry

Day 14

Breakfast-Scrambled Eggs

Lunch- Simple Pizza Rolls

Dinner- Lemon Dill Trout

Day 15

Breakfast-Strawberry Protein Smoothie

Lunch-Bacon and Zucchini Noodles Salad

Dinner-Spinach Soup

The list of food items in this meal plan is not exhaustive. You can change the menu as per the availability of the products.

If you wish to avoid your breakfast or any other meal in order to practice fasting, then you are supposed to keep drinking water in that period of time and also make sure that you take multi-vitamins prescribed by a physician.

Following provided is a list of foods that you can take while on intermittent fasting inspired keto diet-

1. Vegetables
2. Proteins
3. Oil and good fats
4. Beverages
5. Seeds and nuts
6. Diary

The list of foods provided under are to be completely avoided or should be taken in a minimal amount-

1. Processed Foods
2. Artificial Sweeteners
3. Alcohol
4. Milk
5. Refined fats
6. Legumes
7. Soy Products
8. Grains

Chapter 7- Breakfast Recipes

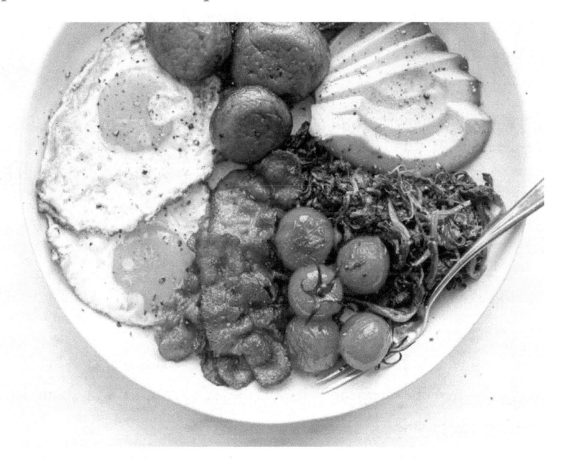

7.1 Delicious Poached Eggs
Ready in about 45 minutes | Servings-4 | Difficulty- Easy

Ingredients

- Three minced garlic cloves
- One tablespoon of ghee
- One chopped white onion
- One chopped Serrano pepper
- Salt and black pepper to the taste
- One chopped red bell pepper

- Three chopped tomatoes
- One teaspoon of paprika
- One teaspoon of cumin
- A quarter teaspoon of chili powder
- One tablespoon of chopped cilantro
- Six eggs

Instructions

1. Heat the pan over medium heat with the ghee, add the onion, stir and cook and stir for ten minutes.
2. Add the garlic and Serrano pepper, stir and cook over medium heat for a minute.
3. Add red bell pepper and cook for 10 minutes, stirring and cooking.
4. Add the tomatoes, pepper, salt, chili powder, paprika and cumin, stir and cook for 10 minutes.
5. In the pan, crack the eggs, season them with pepper and salt, cover the pan and cook for another 6 minutes.
6. In the end, sprinkle with cilantro and serve.

7.2 Delicious Eggs and Sausages

Ready in about 45 minutes | Servings-6 | Difficulty- Easy

Ingredient

- Five tablespoons of ghee
- Twelve eggs
- Salt and black pepper as per taste

- One of torn spinach
- Twelve slices of ham
- Two chopped sausages
- One chopped yellow onion
- One chopped red bell pepper

Instructions

1. Heat a saucepan over medium heat with one tablespoon of ghee, add the onion and sausages, stir and cook for five minutes.

2. Add the bell pepper, pepper and salt, stir and cook for an additional three minutes and place in a bowl.

3. Melt and divide the rest of the ghee into 1two cups of cake molds.

4. In each cupcake mold, add a slice of ham, divide each spinach and then the sausage mix.

5. Break an egg on top, place everything in the oven and bake for 20 minutes at 425 ° Fahrenheit

6. Before serving, leave your cupcakes to cool down a bit.

7.3 Delicious Breakfast Bowl

Ready in about 30 minutes | Servings-1 | Difficulty- Easy

Ingredients

- Four ounces of ground beef
- One chopped yellow onion
- Eight sliced mushrooms
- Salt and black pepper as per taste
- Two whisked eggs

- One tablespoon of coconut oil
- Half a teaspoon of teaspoon smoked paprika
- One avocado, pitted, peeled and chopped
- Twelve pitted and sliced black olives

Instructions

1. Heat a saucepan over medium heat with the coconut oil, add the onions, mushrooms, pepper and salt, stir and cook for five minutes.
2. Add the beef and paprika, stir, cook and transfer to a bowl for 10 minutes.
3. Over medium heat, heat the pan again, add the eggs, some pepper and salt and scramble.
4. Put the beef mix back in the pan and stir.
5. Add the olives and avocado, stir, and cook over medium heat for a minute
6. Transfer and serve in a bowl.

7.4 Keto Breakfast Mix

Ready in about 20 minutes | Servings-2 | Difficulty- Easy

Ingredients

- Five tablespoons of unsweetened coconut flakes
- Seven tablespoons of Hemp seeds
- Five tablespoons of Ground Flaxseed
- Two tablespoons of ground Sesame
- Two tablespoons of unsweetened cocoa, dark
- Two tablespoons of Psyllium husk

Instructions:

1. Grind the sesame and the flaxseed. Ensure that you only grind the sesame seeds for a short time.

2. In a jar, mix all the ingredients and shake them well.

3. Keep refrigerated until ready for consumption.

4. Serve softened with black coffee or still water and, if you want to increase your fat intake, add coconut oil. It also combines well with cream or with cheese from mascarpone.

7.5 Pumpkin Pie Keto Spiced Latte

Ready in about 20 minutes | Servings-2 | Difficulty- Easy

Ingredients

- Two cups of strong and freshly brewed coffee

- One cup of Coconut Milk

- A quarter cup of Pumpkin Puree

- Half teaspoon of Cinnamon

- One teaspoon of Vanilla Extract

- Two teaspoons of Pumpkin Pie Spice Blend

- 15 drops of Liquid Stevia

- Two tablespoons of Butter

- Two tablespoons of Heavy Whipping Cream

Instructions

1. Cook the pumpkin, butter, milk and spices over medium-low flame,

2. Add two cups of solid coffee and blend together until bubbling.

3. Remove from the stove, apply cream and stevia, and then whisk together with an electric mixer.

4. Top with whipped cream and enjoy.

7.6 Keto Frittata

Ready in about one hour 10 minutes | Servings-4 | Difficulty- Moderate

Ingredients

- Nine ounces of spinach
- Twelve eggs
- One ounce of pepperoni
- One teaspoon of minced garlic
- Salt and black pepper to the taste
- Five ounces of shredded mozzarella
- Half cup of grated parmesan
- Half cup of ricotta cheese
- Four tablespoons of olive oil
- A pinch of nutmeg

Instructions

1. Squeeze out the spinach liquid and put it in a bowl.
2. Mix the eggs with the salt, nutmeg, pepper, and garlic in another bowl and whisk well.
3. Add the spinach, ricotta and parmesan and whisk well.
4. Pour this into a saucepan, sprinkle on top with mozzarella and pepperoni, place in the oven and bake for 45 minutes at 375 ° Fahrenheit.
5. Leave the frittata for a few minutes to cool down before serving.

7.7 Keto Fall Pumpkin Spiced French Toast

Ready in about 20 minutes | Servings-2 | Difficulty- Easy

Ingredients

- Four slices of Pumpkin Bread
- One large Egg
- Two tablespoons of cream
- Half teaspoon of Vanilla Extract
- 1/8 teaspoon of Orange Extract
- A quarter teaspoon of Pumpkin Pie Spice
- Two tablespoons of butter

Instructions

Cook the pumpkin, butter, milk and spices over a medium-low flame.

Add two cups of solid coffee and blend together until bubbling.

Remove from the stove, apply cream and stevia, and then whisk together with an electric mixer.

Top with whipped cream and serve.

7.8 Scrambled Eggs

Ready in about 20 minutes | Servings-1 | Difficulty- Easy

Ingredients

- Four chopped bell mushrooms
- Three whisked eggs
- Salt and black pepper to the taste
- Two chopped ham slices
- A quarter cup of chopped red bell pepper
- Half cup of chopped spinach

- One tablespoon of coconut oil

Instructions

Heat a saucepan over medium heat with half the oil, add the mushrooms, spinach, bell pepper and ham, stir and simmer for four minutes.

Heat up another pan over medium heat with the rest of the oil, add the eggs and scramble them.

Stir in the vegetables and ham, pepper and salt, stir, simmer and cook for one minute and then serve.

7.9 Feta and Asparagus Delight
Ready in about 35 minutes | Servings-2 | Difficulty- Easy

Ingredients

- Twelve asparagus spears
- One tablespoon of olive oil
- Two chopped green onions
- One minced garlic clove
- Six eggs
- Salt and black pepper to the taste
- Half cup of feta cheese

Instructions

1. Heat a pan over medium heat with some water, add asparagus, stir for eight minutes, drain well, chop two spears and reserve the remainder.

2. Over medium heat, heat a pan with the oil, add the garlic, onions and chopped asparagus, stir and cook for five minutes.

3. Add salt, pepper and eggs, stir, cover and cook for five minutes.

4. On top of your frittata, arrange the whole asparagus, sprinkle with cheese, place in the oven at 350 ° F and bake for nine minutes.

5. Divide and serve between plates.

7.10 Eggs Baked in Avocados

Ready in about 30 minutes | Servings-4 | Difficulty- Easy

Ingredients

- Two avocados, cut in halves and pitted
- Four eggs
- Salt and black pepper to the taste
- One tablespoon of chopped chives

Instructions

1. Scoop some of the avocado halves with some flesh and assemble them in a baking dish.

2. In each avocado, crack an egg, season with pepper and salt, place them at 425 degrees F in the oven and bake for 20 minutes.

3. In the end, sprinkle the chives and serve them for breakfast.

Chapter 8- Lunch Recipes

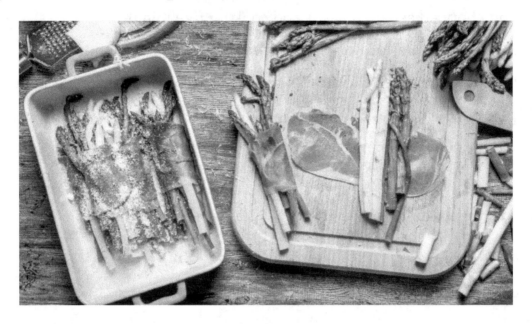

8.1 Lunch Caesar Salad

Ready in about 10 minutes | Servings-2 | Difficulty- Easy

Ingredients

- One pitted, peeled and sliced avocado

- Salt and black pepper to the taste

- Three tablespoons of creamy Caesar dressing

- One cup of cooked and crumbled bacon

- One grilled and shredded chicken breast

Instructions

1. Mix the avocado with the chicken breast and bacon in a salad bowl and stir.

2. Add salt and pepper, Caesar dressing, toss to coat, split into two bowls and serve.

8.2 Keto Lunch Jambalaya

Ready in about 40 minutes | Servings-2 | Difficulty- Moderate

Ingredients

- One medium cauliflower
- One coarsely chopped green pepper
- Two stalks of coarsely chopped celery
- One diced small onion
- Two minced cloves of garlic
- Three cubed boneless chicken breasts
- Eight ounces of sliced smoked sausage
- Eight ounces of ham, cubed
- Fourteen and a half ounce can of diced tomatoes, undrained
- Eight ounce can of tomato sauce
- Three teaspoons of Cajun Seasoning
- Salt and pepper according to taste
- Cooking oil

Instructions

1. Heat two tablespoons of oil in an 8-quart Dutch oven or skillet.
2. On a medium-high flame, sauté the peppers, garlic, chicken, celery, onion and Cajun seasoning until the chicken is almost cooked.
3. Add the cauliflower, ham and sausage. Mix thoroughly.
4. Add the tomato sauce and tomatoes to the mix. Bring it to a simmer, and then turn it back to low.

5. Cover until the cauliflower is moist but not mushy, and cook for around twenty minutes.

6. Season with salt and pepper and then serve after removing from heat.

8.3 Lunch Tacos

Ready in about 40 minutes | Servings-3 | Difficulty- Moderate

Ingredients

- Two cups of grated cheddar cheese
- One small pitted, peeled and chopped avocado
- One cup of cooked favorite taco meat
- Two teaspoons of sriracha sauce
- A quarter cup of chopped tomatoes
- Cooking spray
- Salt and black pepper as per taste

Instructions

1. Spray on a lined baking dish with some cooking oil.

2. Cover on the baking sheet with cheddar cheese, put in the oven at 400 degrees F, and bake for 15 minutes.

3. Spread the taco meat over the cheese and cook for a further 10 minutes.

4. Meanwhile, combine the avocado with tomatoes, sriracha, salt and pepper in a bowl and swirl.

5. Spread this over the layers of taco and cheddar, let the tacos cool down a little, use a pizza slicer to slice and serve for lunch.

8.4 Keto Chicken Enchilada Soup

Ready in about 40 minutes | Servings-3 | Difficulty- Moderate

Ingredients

- Six oz. Shredded chicken
- Two teaspoons of Cumin
- One teaspoon of Oregano
- One teaspoon of Chili Powder
- Half teaspoon of Cayenne Pepper
- Half cup of chopped cilantro
- Half medium Lime, juiced
- three tablespoons of Olive Oil
- Three stalks of diced Celery
- One medium diced Red Bell Pepper, diced
- Two teaspoons of garlic, minced
- Four cups of Chicken Broth
- One cup of Diced Tomatoes
- Eight oz. of Cream Cheese

Instructions

1. Heat the oil in a pan and add the celery and pepper. Add the tomatoes and cook for 2-3 minutes once the celery is soft.
2. Add the spices to the pan and mix well.
3. Add the chicken broth and the cilantro to the mixture, boil, and then reduce to low for 20 minutes to simmer.
4. Then add the cream cheese and bring it back to the boil. Once it has cooked, reduce the heat to low and cover and cook for 25 minutes.
5. Scrap the chicken and add it to the pot, then top it with half the lime juice.

6. Mix together everything.

7. Serve with coriander, sour cream or shredded cheese.

8.5 Simple Pizza Rolls

Ready in about 40 minutes | Servings-6 | Difficulty- Moderate

Ingredients

- A quarter cups of chopped mixed red and green bell peppers
- Two cups of shredded mozzarella cheese
- One teaspoon of pizza seasoning
- Two tablespoons of chopped onion
- One chopped tomato
- Salt and black pepper to the taste
- A quarter cups of pizza sauce
- Half cup of crumbled and cooked sausage

Instructions

1. On a lined and lightly oiled baking dish, spread mozzarella cheese, sprinkle pizza seasoning on top, put at 400 °F in the oven and bake for 20 minutes.

2. Spread the sausage, onion, tomatoes and bell pepper all over and drizzle the tomato sauce at the top. Taking the pizza crust out of the oven.

3. Place them back in the oven and bake for ten more minutes.

4. Take the pizza from the oven, leave it aside for a few minutes, break it into six pieces, roll each slice and eat it for lunch.

8.6 Lunch Stuffed Peppers

Ready in about 50 minutes | Servings-4 | Difficulty- Moderate

Ingredients

- Four big banana peppers cut into halves lengthwise
- One tablespoon of ghee
- Salt and black pepper to the taste
- Half teaspoon of herbs de Provence
- One pound of chopped sweet sausage
- Three tablespoons of chopped yellow onions
- Some marinara sauce
- A drizzle of olive oil

Instructions

1. Season the banana peppers with pepper and salt, drizzle with the oil, rub well and bake for 20 minutes in the oven at 325 ° F.
2. Meanwhile, over medium, prepare, heat a skillet, add the pieces of sausage, mix and cook for 5 minutes.
3. Combine the onion, herbs, salt, pepper and ghee, mix well and simmer for 5 minutes.
4. Take the peppers out of the oven, load them with the sausage mix, place them in a dish that is oven-proof, drizzle them with the marinara sauce, placed them back in the oven and bake for another 10 minutes.
5. Serve and enjoy.

8.7 Special Lunch Burgers

Ready in about 35 minutes | Servings-8 | Difficulty- Moderate

Ingredients

- One pound ground brisket
- One pound ground beef

- Salt and black pepper as per taste

- Eight butter slices

- One tablespoon of minced garlic

- One tablespoon of Italian seasoning

- Two tablespoons of mayonnaise

- One tablespoon of ghee

- Two tablespoons of olive oil

- One chopped yellow onion

- One tablespoon of water

Instructions

1. Mix the beef, pepper, salt, Italian herbs, mayo and garlic with the brisket in a bowl and stir well.

2. Form 8 patties into each one to create a pocket.

3. With butter-slices, stuff each burger and seal it.

4. Over medium pressure, heat the pan with the oil, add the onions, stir and simmer for 2 minutes.

5. Apply the water, swirl and pick them up in the pan corner.

6. Put the burgers with the onions in the pan and cook them for ten minutes over moderate flame.

7. Flip them over, apply the ghee, and simmer for ten more minutes.

8. Break the burgers into buns and place them on top of caramelized onions.

8.8 Keto Roasted Pepper and Cauliflower

Ready in about 50 minutes | Servings-4 | Difficulty- Moderate

Ingredients

- Two halved and de-seeded Red Bell Peppers
- Half head of cauliflower cut into florets
- Two tablespoons of Duck Fat
- Three medium diced green Onions
- Three cups of Chicken Broth
- Half cup Heavy Cream
- Four tablespoons of Duck Fat
- Salt and pepper as per taste
- One teaspoon of Garlic Powder
- One teaspoon of Dried Thyme
- One teaspoon of Smoked Paprika
- A quarter teaspoon of Red Pepper Flakes
- Four oz. Goat Cheese

Instructions

1. Preheat the oven to 400 °F

Clean, de-seed, and half-slice the peppers

Broil until the flesh is burnt and blackened for about 10-15 minutes.

Place in a container with a cover to steam when finished cooking cauliflower.

Sprinkle two tablespoons of melted duck fat, pepper and salt into sliced cauliflower florets.

Cook for 30-35 minutes in the oven.

Pick off the skins of the peppers by gently peeling them off.

Heat Four tablespoons of duck fat in a pot and add the diced green onion.

To toast, apply seasonings to the plate, then add red pepper, chicken broth, and cauliflower to the skillet.

For 10-20 minutes, let this boil.

Bring the mixture to an immersion blender. Make sure that it emulsifies both fats.

Then apply the cream and combine.

Serve with some bacon and goats' cheese. Add thyme and green onion to garnish.

8.9 Bacon and Zucchini Noodles Salad
Ready in about 10 minutes | Servings-2 | Difficulty- Easy

Ingredients

- One cup of baby spinach
- Four cups of zucchini noodles
- 1/3 cups of crumbled bleu cheese
- 1/3 cups of thick cheese dressing
- Half cup of cooked and crumbled bacon
- Black pepper as per taste

Instructions

1. Mix the spinach with the bacon, zucchini noodles and the bleu cheese in a salad dish, and toss.
2. Apply the black pepper and cheese dressing as per taste, toss well to cover, distribute into two bowls and eat.

8.10 Keto Slow Cooker Buffalo Chicken Soup
Ready in about 6 hours and 20 minutes | Servings-2 | Difficulty- Hard

Ingredients

- Three Chicken Thighs, de-boned and sliced
- One teaspoon of Onion Powder
- One teaspoon of Garlic Powder
- Half teaspoon Celery Seed
- A quarter cup of butter
- Half cup of Frank's Hot Sauce
- Three cups of Beef Broth
- One cup of Heavy Cream
- Two oz. Cream Cheese
- A quarter teaspoon of Xanthan Gum
- Salt and pepper as per taste

Instructions

1. Begin by de-boning the chicken thighs, break the chicken into chunks and place the remainder of the ingredients in a slow cooker in the crockpot with the exception of cream, cheese, and xanthan gum.

2. Set a low, slow cooker for 6 hours (or a high one for 3 hours) and cook fully.

3. Remove the chicken from the slow cooker until it is done, and shred it with a fork.

4. Using the slow cooker to combine cream, cheese, and xanthan gum. Combine it all together

5. Transfer the chicken to the slow cooker and blend.

6. Season it with salt, pepper, and hot sauce. Serve.

Chapter 9- Dinner Recipes

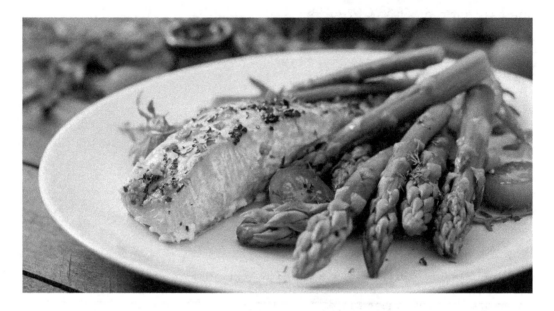

9.1 Buffalo Blue Cheese Chicken Wedges

Ready in about 40 minutes | Servings-2 | Difficulty-Moderate

Ingredients

- One head of lettuce
- Bleu cheese dressing
- Two tablespoons of crumbled blue cheese
- Four strips of bacon
- Two boneless chicken breasts
- 3/4 cup of any buffalo sauce

Instructions

1. Boil a big pot of salted water.
2. Add two chicken breasts to the water and simmer for 30 minutes, or until the internal temperature of the chicken reaches 180 °C.
3. Let the chicken rest for 10 minutes to cool.

4. Take apart the chicken into strips using a fork.

5. Cook and cool bacon strips, crumble reserve,

6. Merge the scrapped chicken and buffalo sauce over medium heat, then mix until warm.

7. Break the lettuce into wedges and apply the appropriate amount of blue cheese dressing to it.

8. Add crumbles of blue cheese.

9. Add the chicken-pulled buffalo.

10. Cover with more crumbles of blue cheese and fried crumbled bacon.

11. Serve.

9.2 Cauliflower Bread Garlic sticks

Ready in about 55 minutes | Servings-2 | Difficulty-Moderate

Ingredients

- Two cups of cauliflower rice
- One tablespoon of organic butter
- Three teaspoons of minced garlic
- A quarter teaspoon of red pepper flakes
- Half teaspoon of Italian seasoning
- 1/8 teaspoon of kosher salt
- One cup of shredded mozzarella cheese
- One egg
- One cup of grated parmesan cheese

Instructions

1. Preheat the oven to 350° F.

2. Sauté the red pepper flakes and garlic for nearly three minutes and transfer to a bowl of cooked cauliflower. Melt the butter in a small skillet over low heat.

3. Mix the Italian seasoning and salt together.

4. Afterward, refrigerate for 10 minutes.

5. Add the mozzarella cheese and egg to the cauliflower mixture until slightly cooled.

6. A creamy paste in a thin layer lined with parchment paper on a thinly oiled 9-9 baking dish.

7. Bake for thirty minutes.

8. Remove from the oven and finish with a little more parmesan and mozzarella cheese.

9. Put them back in the oven and cook for an extra 8 minutes.

10. Remove from the oven and slice into sticks of the appropriate duration.

9.3 Tasty Baked Fish

Ready in about 40 minutes | Servings-4 | Difficulty-Moderate

Ingredients

- One pound of haddock
- Three teaspoons of water
- Two tablespoons of lemon juice
- Salt and black pepper as per taste
- Two tablespoons of mayonnaise
- One teaspoon of dill weed
- Cooking spray
- A pinch of old bay seasoning

Instructions

1. With some cooking oil, spray a baking dish.

2. Apply the lemon juice, fish and water and toss to cover a little bit.

3. Apply salt, pepper, seasoning with old bay and dill weed and mix again.

4. Add mayonnaise and spread evenly.

5. Place it at 350 ° F in the oven and bake for thirty minutes.

6. Split and serve on a plate.

9.4 Spinach Soup

Ready in about 25 minutes | Servings-8 | Difficulty-Easy

Ingredients

*   Two tablespoons of ghee

*   Twenty ounces of chopped spinach

*   One teaspoon of minced garlic

*   Salt and black pepper as per taste

*   Forty-five ounces of chicken stock

*   Half teaspoons of nutmeg, ground

*   Two cups of heavy cream

*   One chopped yellow onion

Instructions

1. Heat a pot over medium heat with the ghee, add the onion, stir and simmer for 4 minutes.

2. Stir in the garlic, stir and simmer for a minute.

3. Add spinach and stock and simmer for 5 minutes.

4. Blend the broth with an immersion mixer and reheat the soup.

5. Stir in pepper, nutmeg, salt, and cream, stir and simmer for a further 5 minutes.

6. Ladle it into cups and serve.

9.5 Tossed Brussel Sprout Salad

Ready in about 30 minutes | Servings-2 | Difficulty-Easy

Ingredients

- Six Brussels sprouts
- Half teaspoon of apple cider vinegar
- One teaspoon of olive/grapeseed oil
- A quarter teaspoon of salt
- A quarter teaspoon of pepper
- One tablespoon of freshly grated parmesan

Instructions

1. Break and clean Brussels sprouts in half lengthwise, root on, then cut thin slices through them in the opposite direction.

2. Cut the roots and remove them until chopped.

3. Toss the apple cider, oil, pepper and salt together.

4. Sprinkle, blend and eat with your parmesan cheese.

9.6 Special Fish Pie

Ready in about One hour 20 minutes | Servings-6 | Difficulty-Moderate

Ingredients

- One chopped red onion
- Two skinless and medium sliced salmon fillets

- Two skinless and medium sliced mackerel fillets
- Three medium sliced haddock fillets
- Two bay leaves
  - A quarter cup and two tablespoons of ghee
  - One cauliflower head, florets separated
  - Four eggs
  - Four cloves
  - One cup of whipping cream
  - Half cup of water
  - A pinch of nutmeg
  - One teaspoon of Dijon mustard
  - One and a half cup of shredded cheddar cheese
  - A handful of chopped parsley
  - Salt and black pepper as per taste
  - Four tablespoons of chopped chives

Instructions

1. In a saucepan, place some water, add some salt, bring to a boil over medium heat, add the eggs, simmer for ten minutes, heat off, drain, cool, peel and break into quarters.

2. Place the water in another kettle, bring it to a boil, add the florets of cauliflower, simmer for 10 minutes, rinse, add a quarter of a cup of ghee, add it to the mixer, blend properly, and place it in a bowl.

3. Add the cream and half a cup of water to a saucepan, add the fish, toss and cover over medium heat.

4. Put to a boil, reduce heat to a minimum, and steam for 10 minutes. Put the cloves, onion, and bay leave.

5. Take the heat off, put the fish and set it aside in a baking dish.

6. Heat the saucepan with the fish, add the nutmeg, combine and simmer for 5 minutes.

7. Remove from the oven, discard the bay leaves and cloves and blend well with one cup of cheddar cheese and two tablespoons of ghee.

8. On top of the fish, set the egg quarters in the baking dish.

9. Sprinkle with cream and cheese sauce on top of the remaining cheddar cheese, chives and parsley, cover with cauliflower mash, sprinkle with the remaining cheddar cheese, and place in the oven for 30 minutes at 400 ° F.

10. Leave the pie until it is about to slice and serve, to cool down a little.

9.7 Lemon Dill Trout

Ready in about 20 minutes | Servings-4 | Difficulty-Easy

Ingredients

- Two pounds of pan-dressed trout (or other small fish), fresh or frozen
- One and a half teaspoons of salt
- A quarter teaspoon of pepper
- Half cup of butter or margarine
- Two tablespoons of dill weed
- Three tablespoons of lemon juice

Instructions

1. Cut fish lengthwise and season its inside with pepper and salt.

2. With melted butter and dill weed, prepare a frying pan.

3. For about two to three minutes per side, fry the fish flesh side down.

4. Remove the fish.

5. Add lemon juice to butter and dill to create a sauce.

6. Serve the fish and sauce together.

9.8 Sage N Orange Breast of Duck

Ready in about 20 minutes | Servings-4 | Difficulty-Easy

Ingredients

- Six oz. Duck Breast (~6 oz.)

- Two tablespoons of Butter

- One tablespoon of Heavy Cream

- One tablespoon of Swerve

- Half teaspoon of Orange Extract

- A quarter teaspoon of Sage

- One cup of spinach

Instructions

1. Score the duck skin on top of the breast and season with pepper and salt.

2. Brown butter in a saucepan over medium-low heat, and swerve.

3. Add the extract of sage and orange and cook until it is deep orangey in color.

4. Sear duck breasts for few minutes until nicely crunchy.

5. Flip the Breast of the Duck.

6. Add the orange and sage butter to the heavy cream and pour it over the duck.

7. Cook until finished.

8. In the pan that you used to make the sauce, add the spinach and serve with the duck.

9.9 Salmon with Caper Sauce

Ready in about 30 minutes | Servings-3 | Difficulty-Easy

Ingredients

- Three salmon fillets
- Salt and black pepper as per taste
- One tablespoon of olive oil
- One tablespoon of Italian seasoning
- Two tablespoons of capers
- Three tablespoons of lemon juice
- Four minced garlic cloves
- Two tablespoons of ghee

Instructions

1. Heat the olive oil pan over medium heat, add the skin of the fish fillets side by side, season with pepper salt and Italian seasoning, cook for two minutes, toss and cook for another two minutes, remove from heat, cover and leave aside for 15 minutes.
2. Put the fish on a plate and leave it aside.
3. Over medium heat, heat the same pan, add the capers, garlic and lemon juice, stir and cook for two minutes.
4. Remove the heat from the pan, add ghee and stir very well.
5. Put the fish back in the pan and toss with the sauce to coat.
6. Divide and serve on plates.

9.10 Bok Choy Stir Fry

Ready in about 20 minutes | Servings-2 | Difficulty-Easy

Ingredients

- Two minced garlic cloves
- Two cups of chopped bok choy
- Two chopped bacon slices
- Salt and black pepper to the taste
- A drizzle of avocado oil

Instructions

1. Heat a pan over medium heat with the oil, add the bacon, stir and brown until crunchy, move to paper towels and drain the oil.
2. Return the saucepan to medium heat, stir in the garlic and bok choy, and cook for 4 minutes.
3. Stir in salt, pepper and bacon, stir, cook for another 1 minute, divide among plates and serve.

Chapter 10- Appetizer and Snacks Recipes

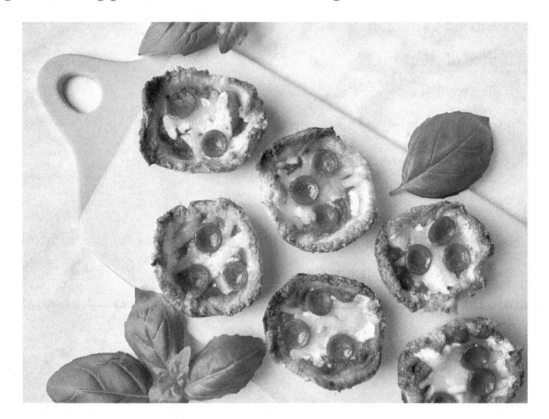

10.1 Cheeseburger Muffins

Ready in about 40 minutes | Servings-9 | Difficulty-Easy

Ingredients

- Half cups of flaxseed meal

- Half cups of almond flour

- Salt and black pepper to the taste

- Two eggs

- One teaspoon of baking powder

- A quarter cups of sour cream

For the filling

- Half teaspoons of onion powder
- Sixteen ounces of ground beef
- Salt and black pepper to the taste
- Two tablespoons of tomato paste
- Half teaspoons of garlic powder
- Half cups of grated cheddar cheese
- Two tablespoons of mustard

Instructions

1. Mix the almond flour with the flaxseed meal, pepper, salt and baking powder in a bowl and whisk together.
2. Add the sour cream and eggs and stir very well.
3. Divide it into a greased muffin pan and use your fingers to press well.
4. Over medium-high heat, heat a pan, add beef, stir and brown for a couple of minutes.
5. Stir well and add pepper, salt, garlic powder, onion powder and tomato paste.
6. Cook for an additional 5 minutes and take the heat off.
7. Fill the crusts with this mixture, place them in the oven at 350 degrees F and bake for fifteen minutes
8. Spread the cheese on top, put it in the oven again and cook the muffins for another 5 minutes.
9. Serve with mustard and your preferred toppings.

10.2 Pesto Crackers

Ready in about 30 minutes | Servings-6 | Difficulty-Easy

Ingredients

- Half teaspoons of baking powder

- Salt and black pepper to the taste

- One and a quarter cups of almond flour

- A quarter teaspoon of basil, dried

- One minced garlic clove

- Two tablespoons of basil pesto

- A pinch of cayenne pepper

- Three tablespoons of ghee

Instructions

1. Mix the pepper, salt, almond flour and baking powder together in a bowl.

2. Stir in the garlic, basil and cayenne.

3. Add whisk the pesto.

4. Also, add ghee and with your finger, mix your dough.

5. Spread this dough on a baking sheet and bake it at 325 degrees F in the oven for 17 minutes.

6. Leave your crackers aside to cool down, cut them and serve.

10.3 Tomato Tarts

Ready in about One hour and 20 minutes | Servings-4 | Difficulty-Easy

Ingredients

- A quarter cups of olive oil

- Two sliced tomatoes

- Salt and black pepper to the taste

For the base

- Five tablespoons of ghee
- One tablespoon psyllium husk
- Half cups of almond flour
- Two tablespoons of coconut flour
- A pinch of salt

For the filling

- Two teaspoons of minced garlic
- Three teaspoons of chopped thyme
- Two tablespoons of olive oil
- Three ounces of crumbled goat cheese
- One small thinly sliced onion

Instructions

1. On a lined baking sheet, spread the tomato slices, season with pepper and salt, drizzle with a quarter of a cup of olive oil, place in the oven at 425 degrees F and bake for 40 minutes.
2. Meanwhile, mix psyllium husk with almond flour, coconut flour, pepper, salt and cold butter in your food processor and stir until you've got your dough.
3. Divide this dough into cupcake molds of silicone, press well, place it in the oven at 350 degrees F and bake for 20 minutes.
4. Remove the cupcakes from the oven and leave them aside.
5. Also, take slices of tomatoes from the oven and cool them down a bit.
6. On top of the cupcakes, divide the tomato slices.

7. Heat a saucepan over medium-high heat with two tablespoons of olive oil, add the onion, stir and cook for 4 minutes.

8. Add the thyme and garlic, stir, cook for another 1 minute and remove from the heat.

9. Spread the mix over the tomato slices.

10. Sprinkle with the goat cheese, put it back in the oven and cook for five more minutes at 350 degrees F.

11. Arrange and serve on a platter.

10.4 Pepper Nachos

Ready in about 30 minutes | Servings-6 | Difficulty-Easy

Ingredients

- One pound of halved mini bell peppers
- Salt and black pepper as per the taste
- One teaspoon of garlic powder
- One teaspoon of sweet paprika
- Half teaspoons of dried oregano
- A quarter teaspoon of red pepper flakes
- One pound of ground beef meat
- One and a half cups of shredded cheddar cheese
- One tablespoon of chili powder
- One teaspoon of ground cumin
- Half cups of chopped tomato
- Sour cream for serving

Instructions

1. Mix the chili powder, pepper, salt, paprika, oregano, cumin, flakes of pepper and garlic powder in a bowl and stir.

2. Over medium heat, heat a pan, add beef, mix and brown for 10 minutes.

3. Add the mixture of chili powder, stir and take the heat off.

4. On a lined baking sheet, arrange the pepper halves, stuff them with the beef mix, sprinkle the cheese, place in the oven at 400 degrees F and cook for 10 minutes.

5. Remove the peppers from the oven, sprinkle with the tomatoes and divide among the plates and serve with sour cream.

10.5 Pumpkin Muffins

Ready in about One hour 25 minutes | Servings-18 | Difficulty-Easy

Ingredients

- A quarter cups of sunflower seed butter
- 3/4 cups of pumpkin puree
- Two tablespoons of flaxseed meal
- A quarter cups of coconut flour
- Half cup of erythritol
- Half teaspoons of ground nutmeg
- one teaspoon of ground cinnamon
- Half teaspoons of baking soda
- One egg
- Half teaspoons of baking powder
- A pinch of salt

Instructions

1. Mix the butter with the pumpkin puree and egg in a bowl and mix well.

2. Stir well and add coconut flour, flaxseed meal, erythritol, baking powder, baking soda, nutmeg, cinnamon and a pinch of salt.

3. Spoon this into an oiled muffin pan, add in the oven at 350 degrees F and cook for 15 minutes.

4. Let the muffins cool and serve them as a snack.

10.6 Fried Queso

Ready in about One hour 20 minutes | Servings-6 | Difficulty-Easy

Ingredients

- Two ounces of pitted and chopped olives,

- Five ounces of cubed and freeze queso Blanco

- A pinch of red pepper flakes

- One and a half tablespoons of olive oil

Instructions

1. Over medium-high heat, heat a pan with the oil, add cheese cubes and fry until the lower part melts a bit.

2. Flip the spatula cubes and sprinkle on top with black olives.

3. Let the cubes cook a little more, flip and sprinkle with the red flakes of pepper and cook until crispy.

4. Flip, cook until crispy on the other side, then move to a chopping board, cut into tiny blocks, and then serve.

10.7 Tortilla Chips

Ready in about 25 minutes | Servings-6 | Difficulty-Easy

Ingredients

For the tortillas

- Two teaspoons of olive oil
- One cup of flaxseed meal
- Two tablespoons of psyllium husk powder
- A quarter teaspoon of xanthan gum
- One cup of water
- Half teaspoons of curry powder
- Three teaspoons of coconut flour

For the chips

- Six flaxseed tortillas
- Salt and black pepper to the taste
- Three tablespoons of vegetable oil
- Fresh salsa for serving
- Sour cream for serving

Instructions

1. Combine psyllium powder, flaxseed meal, xanthan gum, olive oil curry powder and water in a bowl and mix until an elastic dough is obtained.
2. On a working surface, spread coconut flour.
3. Divide the dough into six pieces, place each portion on the work surface, roll it into a circle and cut it into six pieces each.
4. Over medium-high heat, heat a pan with vegetable oil, add tortilla chips, cook on each side for 2 minutes and transfer to paper towels.
5. Put in a bowl of tortilla chips, season with pepper and salt and serve on the side with sour cream and fresh salsa.

10.8 Jalapeno Balls

Ready in about One hour 20 minutes | Servings-3 | Difficulty-Easy

Ingredients

- Three slices of bacon
- Three ounces of cream cheese
- A quarter teaspoon of onion powder
- Salt and black pepper as per taste
- One chopped jalapeno pepper
- Half teaspoons of dried parsley
- A quarter teaspoon of garlic powder

Instructions

1. Over medium-high heat, heat a skillet, add bacon, cook until crispy, switch to paper towels, remove the fat and crumble.
2. Reserve the pan's bacon fat.
3. Combine the jalapeno pepper, cream cheese, garlic powder and onion, parsley, pepper and salt in a bowl and stir thoroughly.
4. Use this blend to mix bacon crumbles and bacon fat, stir softly, form balls, and serve.

10.9 Maple and Pecan Bars

Ready in about 40 minutes | Servings-12 | Difficulty-Easy

Ingredients

- Half cups of flaxseed meal
- two cups of pecans, toasted and crushed

- one cup of almond flour
- Half cups of coconut oil
- A quarter teaspoon of stevia
- Half cups of coconut, shredded
- A quarter cups of maple syrup
- **For the maple syrup**
- A quarter cups of erythritol
- Two and a quarter teaspoons of coconut oil
- One tablespoon of ghee
- A quarter teaspoon of xanthan gum
- 3/4 cups of water
- Two teaspoons of maple extract
- Half teaspoons of vanilla extract

Instructions

1. Combine ghee with two and a quarter teaspoons of xanthan gum and coconut oil in a heat-proof bowl, stir, put in your oven and heat up for 1 minute.
2. Add the extract of erythritol, water, maple and vanilla, mix well and fire for 1 minute more in the microwave.
3. Mix the flaxseed meal and the coconut and almond flour in a bowl and stir.
4. Add the pecans, and stir them again.
5. Apply a quarter of a cup of maple syrup, stevia, and half a cup of coconut oil, and mix well.
6. Spread this in a baking dish, push well, position it at 350 degrees F in the oven and cook for 25 minutes.

7. To cool off, leave it aside, break into 12 bars and act as a keto snack.

10.10 Broccoli and Cheddar Biscuits

Ready in about One hour 35 minutes | Servings-12 | Difficulty-Easy

Ingredients

- Four cups of broccoli florets

- One and a half cups of almond flour

- One teaspoon of paprika

- Salt and black pepper to the taste

- Two eggs

- A quarter cup of coconut oil

- Two cups of grated cheddar cheese

- One teaspoon of garlic powder

- Half teaspoons of apple cider vinegar

- Half teaspoons of baking soda

Instructions

1. In your food processor, place the broccoli florets, add some pepper and salt and combine well.

2. Mix pepper, salt, paprika, baking soda and garlic powder with almond flour in a bowl and stir.

3. Apply the coconut oil, cheddar cheese, vinegar and eggs and stir.

4. Attach the broccoli and stir some more.

5. Shape Twelve patties, arrange them on a baking sheet, put them at 375 degrees F in the oven and bake for 20 minutes.

6. Switch the broiler in the oven and broil the biscuits for another 5 minutes.

7. Arrange and serve on a platter.

Chapter 11- Dessert Recipes

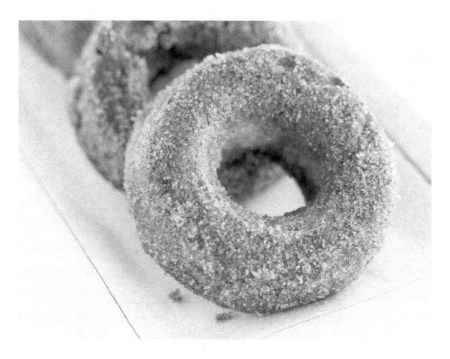

11.1 Chocolate Truffles

Ready in about 20 minutes | Servings-22 | Difficulty-Easy

Ingredients

- One cup of sugar-free chocolate chips
- Two tablespoons of butter
- 2/3 cups of heavy cream
- Two teaspoons of brandy
- Two tablespoons of swerve
- A quarter teaspoon of vanilla extract
- Cocoa powder

Instructions

1. In a fire-proof mug, add heavy cream, swerve, chocolate chips and butter, stir, put in the microwave and heat for 1 minute.

2. Leave for 5 minutes, blend well, and combine with the vanilla and the brandy.

3. Stir again. Set aside for a few hours in the fridge.

4. Shape the truffles using a melon baller, cover them in cocoa powder and then serve them.

11.2 Keto Doughnuts

Ready in about 25 minutes | Servings-24 | Difficulty-Easy

Ingredients

- A quarter cups of erythritol
- A quarter cups of flaxseed meal
- 3/4 cups of almond flour
- One teaspoon of baking powder
- One teaspoon of vanilla extract
- Two eggs
- Three tablespoons of coconut oil
- A quarter cups of coconut milk
- Twenty drops of red food coloring
- A pinch of salt
- One tablespoon of cocoa powder

Instructions

1. Mix together the almond flour, cocoa powder, baking powder, erythritol and salt in a bowl and stir.

2. Mix the coconut oil with vanilla, coconut milk, food coloring and eggs in another bowl and stir.

3. Mix mixtures, use a hand mixer to stir, move to a bag, cut a hole in the bag and shape a baking sheet with 12 doughnuts.

4. Place it in the oven at 350 degrees F and cook for 15 minutes.

5. On a tray, place them and eat them.

11.3 Chocolate Bombs

Ready in about 20 minutes | Servings-12 | Difficulty-Easy

Ingredients

- Ten tablespoons of coconut oil
- Three tablespoons of chopped macadamia nuts
- Two packets of stevia
- Five tablespoons of unsweetened coconut powder
- A pinch of salt

Instructions

1. Place coconut oil in a casserole dish and melt over medium heat.

2. Apply stevia, salt and cocoa powder, mix well and remove from the heat.

3. Spoon this into a tray of candy and store it for a while in the freezer.

4. Sprinkle the macadamia nuts on top and hold them in the refrigerator until served.

11.4 Simple and Delicious Mousse

Ready in about 10 minutes | Servings-12 | Difficulty-Easy

Ingredients

- Eight ounces of mascarpone cheese

- 3/4 teaspoons of vanilla stevia

- One cup of whipping cream

- Half-pint of blueberries

- Half-pint of strawberries

Instructions

1. Combine the whipped cream with mascarpone and stevia in a cup and blend well with your mixer.

2. Assemble twelve glasses with a coating of strawberries and blueberries, then a layer of milk, and so on.

3. Serve cool.

11.5 Strawberry Pie

Ready in about 2 hours and 20 minutes | Servings-12 | Difficulty-Hard

Ingredients

For the filling

- One teaspoon of gelatin

- Eight ounces of cream cheese

- Four ounces of strawberries

- Two tablespoons of water

- Half tablespoon of lemon juice

- A quarter teaspoon of stevia

- Half cups of heavy cream

- Eight ounces of chopped strawberries for serving

- Sixteen ounces of heavy cream for serving

For the crust

- One cup of shredded coconut

- One cup of sunflower seeds

- A quarter cup of butter

- A pinch of salt

Instructions

1. Mix the sunflower seeds with coconut, butter and a pinch of salt in your food processor and stir well.

2. Place this in a greased springform pan and push the bottom well.

3. Heat a skillet over medium heat with the water, add gelatin, mix until it dissolves, remove the heat and leave to cool off.

4. Add it to your food processor, mix and blend well with 4 ounces of cream cheese, lemon juice, strawberries and stevia.

5. Stir well, pour half a cup of heavy cream and scatter over the crust.

6. Before slicing and serving, top with 8 ounces of strawberries and 16 ounces of heavy cream and keep in the refrigerator for 2 hours.

11.6 Keto Cheesecakes

Ready in about 25 minutes | Servings-9 | Difficulty-Easy

Ingredients

For the cheesecakes

- Two tablespoons of butter

- Eight ounces of cream cheese

- Three tablespoons of coffee
- Three eggs
- 1/3 cups of swerve
- One tablespoon of sugar-free caramel syrup

For the frosting

- Three tablespoons of sugar-free caramel syrup
- Three tablespoons of butter
- Eight ounces of soft mascarpone cheese
- Two tablespoons of swerve

Instructions

1. Combine eggs with cream cheese, two tablespoons butter, one tablespoon caramel syrup, coffee, and 1/3 cup swerve in your blender and pulse very well.

2. Spoon this into a pan of cupcakes, place it at 350 degrees F in the oven and cook for 15 minutes.

3. To cool down, leave aside and then keep in the freezer for three hours.

4. Meanwhile, mix three tablespoons butter with three tablespoons caramel syrup, two tablespoons swerve and mascarpone cheese in a bowl and mix well.

5. Spoon the cheesecakes over and serve them.

11.7 Peanut Butter Fudge

Ready in about 2 hours and 15 minutes | Servings-12 | Difficulty-Hard

Ingredients

- One cup of unsweetened peanut butter
- A quarter cups of almond milk
- Two teaspoons of vanilla stevia
- One cup of coconut oil
- A pinch of salt

For the topping

- Two tablespoons of swerve
- Two tablespoons of melted coconut oil
- A quarter cups of cocoa powder

Instructions

1. Combine peanut butter with one cup of coconut oil in a heat-proof bowl, stir and heat in your microwave until it melts.
2. Add stevia, a pinch of salt and almond milk, mix it well and pour into a lined loaf pan.
3. Keep it for 2 hours in the refrigerator and then slice it.
4. Mix two tablespoons of cocoa powder and melted coconut in a bowl and swirl and stir well.
5. Drizzle over your peanut butter fudge with the sauce and serve.

11.8 Chocolate Pie

Ready in about 3 hours and 30 minutes | Servings-10 | Difficulty-Hard

Ingredients

For the filling

- One tablespoon vanilla extract

- Four tablespoons of sour cream
- One teaspoon of vanilla extract
- Four tablespoons of butter
- Sixteen ounces of cream cheese
- Half cup of cut stevia
- Two teaspoons of granulated stevia
- Half cup of cocoa powder
- One cup of whipping cream

For crust

- Half teaspoons of baking powder
- One and a half cups of the almond crust
- A quarter cup of stevia
- A pinch of salt
- One egg
- One and a half teaspoons of vanilla extract
- Three tablespoons of butter
- One teaspoon of butter for the pan

Instructions

1. With one teaspoon of butter, oil a springform pan and leave aside for now.

2. Mix the baking powder with a quarter cup of stevia, almond flour and a pinch of salt in a bowl and stir.

3. Add three tablespoons of butter, one teaspoon of egg, and one and a half teaspoons of vanilla extract, then mix till the time the dough is ready.

4. Press it well into the springform pan, place it at 375 degrees F in the oven and cook it for 11 minutes.

5. Take the pie crust out of the oven, cover it with tin foil and cook for another 8 minutes.

6. Take it out of the oven again and set it aside to cool down.

7. Meanwhile, add sour cream, four tablespoons of butter, one tablespoon of vanilla extract, half a cup of cocoa powder and stevia to the cream cheese in a bowl and mix it well.

8. Mix two teaspoons of stevia and one teaspoon of vanilla extract with the whipping cream in another bowl and stir using your mixer.

9. Combine two mixtures, pour into the pie crust, spread well, place for 3 hours in the refrigerator and serve.

11.9 Raspberry and Coconut Dessert

Ready in about 20 minutes | Servings-12 | Difficulty-Easy

Ingredients

- Half cup of coconut butter
- Half cup of coconut oil
- Half cup of dried raspberries
- A quarter cups of swerve
- Half cup of shredded coconut

Instructions

1. Mix the dried berries in your food processor very well.

2. Heat a pan over medium heat with the butter.

3. Stir in the coconut, oil and swerve, stir and cook for 5 minutes.

4. Pour half of this and spread well into a lined baking pan.

5. Add raspberry powder and also spread.

6. Spread the rest of the butter mix on top and keep it in the fridge for a while.

7. Cut and serve into pieces.

11.10 Vanilla Ice Cream

Ready in about 3 hours 20 minutes | Servings-6 | Difficulty-Hard

Ingredients

- Four eggs, yolks and whites separated

- A quarter teaspoon of cream of tartar

- Half cups of swerve

- One tablespoon of vanilla extract

- One and a quarter cups of heavy whipping cream

Instructions

1. Mix the egg whites with the tartar cream in a bowl and swerve and swirl using your mixer.

2. Whisk the cream with the vanilla extract in another bowl and mix thoroughly.

3. Combine and gently whisk the two mixtures.

4. Whisk the egg yolks very well in another bowl and then apply the combination of two egg whites.

5. Gently stir, put it into a container and leave it in the refrigerator for 3 hours until the ice cream is eaten.

Chapter 12- Smoothie Recipes

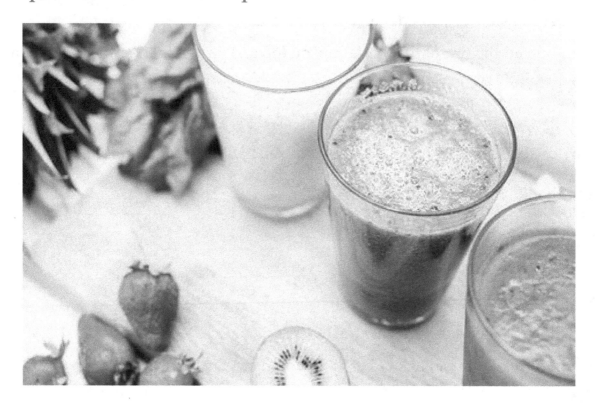

12.1 Minted Iced Berry Sparkler

Ready in about 30 minutes | Servings-2 | Difficulty-Easy

Ingredients

- One cup of mixed frozen berries
- One lime or lemon
- One cup of fresh mint
- Twenty drops liquid Stevia extract (Clear / Berry)
- One large bottle of water
- Ice

Instructions

1. Wash the mint.

2. Cut the lime into wedges that are thin.

3. Using your option of sparkling or still water to put mint, frozen berries, lemon wedges or lime and leftover ingredients into all in a jar.

4. Let yourself relax for 15 minutes or more. The longer you keep it, the taste gets bolder.

5. Serve.

12.2 Body Pumping Smoothie

Ready in about 10 minutes | Servings-2 | Difficulty-Easy

Ingredients

- One beetroot
- One Apple
- Three tablespoons of yogurt
- Handful of mint
- One thumb of a two-inch ginger
- Half teaspoon of black salt or rock salt
- One teaspoon of honey or sugar
- A quarter cup of water

Instructions

1. Clean and remove the beet peel.
2. Slice the medium-sized apple and remove the nuts.
3. Add all the ingredients into the blender.
4. Add ice, then proceed to mix into a paste that is smooth.
5. Add juice from the lemon.
6. Enjoy and serve.

12.3 Kiwi Dream Blender

Ready in about 10 minutes | Servings-2 | Difficulty-Easy

Ingredients

- A quarter average avocado
- One small wedge of Galia melon (or Honeydew, Cantaloupe)
- One scoop of vanilla whey protein powder (vanilla or plain)
- powdered gelatin
- Six drops liquid Stevia extract
- Ice as per the need
- A quarter cups of coconut milk (or coconut cream or full-fat cream)
- A quarter cup of kiwi berries or kiwi fruit
- One tablespoon of chia seeds (or psyllium)
- Half cups of water

Instructions

1. Strip and peel the avocado and put it in a blender.
2. Add the kiwi, melon and the remaining ingredients to the flesh.
3. Blend until completely smooth.
4. Serve.

12.4 Keto Smart Banana Blender

Ready in about 10 minutes | Servings-2 | Difficulty-Easy

Ingredients

- One cup of Spinach
- One cup of Banana

- Half cup of water and yogurt

- Two tablespoons of Pomegranate

- Two tablespoons of Almond meal/Almonds

- One teaspoon of Cinnamon powder

- One teaspoon of Vanilla sugar or Honey or Sugar and vanilla extract

- Ice

Instructions

1. Clean the spinach and chop it coarsely.

2. Cut the Banana into medium-sized portions.

3. To make a half-cup of milk, blend two to three tablespoons of yogurt with water.

4. In a blender, mix all ingredients and process until smooth.

5. If the ideal thickness is met, add ice when blending.

6. Then serve.

12.5 Bright Morning Smoothie
Ready in about 15 minutes | Servings-2 | Difficulty-Easy

Ingredients

- Two cups of Washed Spinach

- Two Large Strawberries

- A quarter cup of Lemon Juice or Fresh Squeezed Orange Juice

- Two tablespoons of Chia Seeds or Powder

- One cup of Green Tea

- One cup of Ice

- Four tablespoons of sweetener of choice

Instructions

1. Place all of the ingredients in a mixer.

2. Blend it all until smooth.

3. Let it rest for about 5-10 minutes, then serve.

12.6 Keto Iced Strawberry and Greens

Ready in about 10 minutes | Servings-2 | Difficulty-Easy

Ingredients

- Half cup coconut water

- One cup of ice

- One cup of washed spinach

- Three large strawberries

- Sweetener to taste

Instructions

1. Blend all the ingredients together in a blender until smooth.

2. Let it rest for 5 minutes and then serve chilled.

12.7 Strawberry Lime Ginger Punch

Ready in about 10 minutes | Servings-2 | Difficulty-Easy

Ingredients

- Two cups of water

- Two tablespoons of raw apple cider vinegar

- Three packets of NuStevia or any other sweetener

- Juice of one lime

- Half teaspoon of ginger powder

- Five frozen strawberries

Instructions

1. Blend all the ingredients together in a blender until smooth.

2. Let it rest for 5 minutes and then serve chilled.

12.8 Mexican Comfort Cream

Ready in about 20 minutes | Servings-2 | Difficulty-Easy

Ingredients

- Two handfuls of almonds blanched

- One cup of almond milk (unsweetened)

- One large egg

- Two tablespoons of whole or ground chia seeds

- One tablespoon of lime zest

- One teaspoon of cinnamon powder or one whole cinnamon stick

- Three tablespoons of erythritol or another healthy low-carb sweetener

- Twenty drops of liquid Stevia extract (Clear / Cinnamon)

- Two cups of warm water

Instructions

1. Put in a bowl lime zest, the blanched almonds and cinnamon stick and cover with two teaspoons of hot water.

2. Let it rest for about eight hours or overnight.

3. Remove the lime zest and cinnamon stick after the almonds have been softened and put them in a shallow saucepan.

4. Mix almond milk. Purée until it's really smooth.

5. Steam the mixture and mix cinnamon and sweeteners before it begins to sizzle.

6. Whisk the egg when stirring constantly and pour it gently into the mixture.

7. Stir for a minute or two over the sun.

8. Remove from the heat and add in the seeds of chia.

9. To thicken the remainder.

10. Serve cold and pour in a bottle.

12.9 Strawberry Protein Smoothie

Ready in about 10 minutes | Servings-2 | Difficulty-Easy

Ingredients

- Half cup water
- One cup of ice
- One scoop of strawberry protein powder
- One egg
- Two tablespoons of cream
- Two strawberries

Instructions

1. Blend ice cubes and water together.

2. Apply the egg, powder and strawberries and start blending.

3. Pour in the cream.

4. Blend it again until smooth in a blender.

5. Serve and enjoy.

12.10 Low-Carb Caribbean Cream

Ready in about 2 hours and 10 minutes | Servings-1 | Difficulty-Moderate

Ingredients

- Half cup of unsweetened coconut milk

- A quarter cups of coconut water or water (iced)

- One shot of dark or white rum

- One slice of fresh pineapple

- Five drops of liquid Stevia extract

Instructions

1. In an ice cube tray, freeze the coconut water for 1-2 hours.

2. Blend coconut milk and pineapple until creamy.

3. Add the coconut water ice cubes and rum to the serving bottle.

4. Add the combined solution.

5. Use the pineapple to garnish.

6. Serve and enjoy.

Keto diet Cookbook

Best and easy diet to follow and maintain

Stacey Bell

Table of Contents

Introduction

We as human are all different, the effect of these eating systems can vary from one person to another but with several modifications to them so that they can suit you, there will only be benefits. Unfortunately, there are some individuals who should not attempt these fat loss regiments. If you have any severe health issues, it is mandatory to seek medical advice prior to beginning the new lifestyle, even if you are generally healthy, it is still advisable to consult a professional.

To clarify things even before diving right into the pool of data contained in this book, it is best to understand the difference between IF and the keto diet. IF is not a diet, but a meal planner that is designed to enhance weight loss and other health advantages, the keto diet is a diet that highly restricts carbohydrates and increases the amount of fat that you take so that you can be fuller for longer and be able to make fat your main energy source in the midst of other advantages that will be discussed later on.

The main reason why many doctors and nutritional experts give the "calories in-calories out" advice is that on paper it is simple and direct. They think that excessive calorie intake is the main cause of obesity; thus, the direct way of reversing this is consuming fewer calories. The 'eat less and move more' approach has been done for a very long time, and it simply does not work. The reason is that obesity and excessive weight gain is more of a hormonal imbalance than a calories imbalance. You will learn more about this and how the IF and the ketogenic diet can assist you in correcting this.

By reading this book, you will find a vast amount of information about IF and the ketogenic diet. You will know why and how they work so well and how they can work together to enhance your weight loss experience. You will also know about their benefits and downsides and how to be safe as you practice them.

During intermittent fasting, your body utilizes stubborn fat as it encourages metabolism that results in heat manufacture. This helps preserve muscle mass during weight loss and increases energy levels for keto dieters who want to lose weight and improve their athletic prowess. Combining the scheme of intermittent fasting and the ketogenic diet can lead to more body fat melting than individuals who follows IF but still consume junk food.

It can also increase your body structure as intermittent fasting improves human growth hormone output but at very large proportion. This hormone performs an enormous part in constructing muscles. The human growth hormone helps an individual reducing body fat concentrations and boost lean body and bone mass, according to studies conducted. Working out in a fasted state can result in metabolic adjustments in your muscle cells arising in energy fat burning. The human growth hormone also enables you to recover from injury or even difficult exercise at a quicker pace. It also decreases skin swelling.

The mixture of the two can even affect the aging process in a beneficial way. They cause the process of stem cells to rise. These are like construction blocks for the body as they can be transformed into any cell the body requires, as well as replacing ancient or harmed cells that keep you younger internally for longer. These stem cells can do wonders to old wounds, chronic pain, and much more. This can enhance your life expectaction as your general health is enhanced by balancing blood glucose, reducing swelling, and improving the free radical defense.

It can boost autophagy. This is simply cell cleaning measures. When it starts, your cells migrate through your inner components and remove any harmed or old cells and replace them with fresh ones. It's like an organ upgrade. It decreases inflammation and improves organ life.

There are no cravings, tiredness, and mood changes when exercising the ketogenic diet and intermittent fasting. This is accomplished through constantly small concentrations of blood sugar. This is because your blood sugar concentrations are not increased by fat. You will be prepared to keep small concentrations of blood sugar that can significantly assist individuals with Type 2 diabetes, even get off their drugs.

The liver transforms fat into packets of energy called ketones that are taken into the blood to offer your cells energy. These ketones destroy the ghrelin, the primary hunger hormone. High concentrations of ghrelin leave you famished while ketones decrease hormone concentrations even if your digestive tract does not contain any meals. This means you can stay without eating for a longer period of time and you won't get hungry. Undoubtedly, the ketogenic diet makes fasting much easier for you to do.

Some individuals follow the ketogenic diet integrated with intermittent fasting. This is by observing the ketogenic nutritional laws while also pursuing the trend of intermittent fasting eating. This can have many advantages, including high-fat burning levels, as both are important in using fats for energy over carbohydrates, providing you energy, reducing cholesterol in your body, controlling your blood sugar that can assist manage type 2 diabetes, helping to cope with hunger, and reducing skin inflammation.

For most individuals, combining the two is comfortable and can significantly speed up the fat burning process, making you accomplish your objectives quicker. However, one or the other can be done alone as they have many comparable advantages. Choosing an intermittent fasting unit that fits you is also essential and always makes sure you consume enough of the macro ingredients. Depending on what was in the meals, the functions can be comparatively fine for both. The job performed will be ideal when you mix both of them and will make weight loss much easier for you to do as both operate in distinct aspects but complement each other superbly.

Successful stories

1. Actor.

John Cusack, the actor, is on a completely Keto diet and the majority of his life revolves around his Keto commitment. He is always seen doing physical activities with his wife, and their children. John admits to never ever getting sick. He follows a diet plan that has proven effective as seen from his movies. He is a big believer in the keto diet and the keto lifestyle.

You look good, where did you lose weight? Shusaku, the man in the center, did a diet that was popular in 2015. The year was 2015, and it was one of the worst years that American History would witness. John -John, the football player, hated tofu and chicken. He is a huge meat eater. That was why he implemented a Keto diet. It is a long-term diet, and it is relatively simple to follow. The kind of food you are going to eat will depend on your daily activity and the activity level on the day. The diet also depends on the activity and physical condition. There are those that enter the diet when they are sick. They do it because we feel good and we are looking good.

2. President Donald Trump.

Donald Trump wanted to lose weight. He was so overweight that he needed to take surgical precautions of his heart as he had developed heart problems. He is exploring various ways to take advantage of the positive effects of the Keto diet he is on. Trump was happy with the results that he was getting from the Keto diet. His heart surgeon had no choice but to say, "it is looking good. We are seeing the pounds melting off that boy." Trump said, "I am a believer in the Keto diet."

3. Kathryn Dennis.

Kathy says she has lost 60 pounds and that she hopes to do another 26-pound weight loss in the next year. She wants to get from 240 pounds to 119 pounds.

The girlfriend of professional football player Nate Washington says she went from a size 26 to a size 4, without taking shots of insulin. She decided to do the Keto diet in order to lose weight. She wanted to do the keto diet because of the weight loss, and the other benefits that the diet has to offer.

4. George W. Bush.

George Bush is a very avid Keto supporter. He has recently joined the Keto diet program and has gotten a lot of compliments and also a lot of medical advice. He started the Keto diet after he was diagnosed with coronary artery disease. His doctor told him to do away with food that has a high-fat content like meat and eggs, He was advised to fish, fruits, and vegetables and to do away with the high carb and fat drinks. He was advised to do away with all that has a high carbohydrate content. These include sugar, sugary drinks, potatoes, rice, pasta, and bread. As a result, he began to lose weight rapidly. He does not drink any high carb or fat meal. He does not like drinking any alcohol as he only drinks small quantities of beer once in a while. He can happily say he is enjoying his life on the Keto diet.

5. Shakira

Shakira is a singer. She is from Columbia, and she has Spanish ancestry. At a certain point in her life, she gave birth to her son, Milan. She gained a lot of weight because she wanted to nurse him. She could not give up on her baby. One day, she looked into the mirror, and she did not recognize herself. She realized that she was not happy. She researched on the Internet, and she came across the Keto diet. She went through it, and she did not move from step one to step two. She was determined to do everything properly. She followed what she was told to do, and she fully embraced the Keto lifestyle. She went on a diet with high fat, protein, and low carb content. She lost weight successfully.

6. Serena Williams.

Serena Williams is a tennis player. She is very successful. She is one of the best tennis players in the world, and she is primarily using the keto diet plan. She has been using the Keto diet because of her desire to lose weight. She does not eat any good that is high in carbs; she only eats vegetables, healthy food, fish, and meat. She consumes coconut oil, coconut milk, and salad dressings. She consumes something that has a high-fat content. She only eats one serving of carbs. This is a very good development for people that are trying to lose weight, and people that are trying to improve theirs constantly. Kick-off your new year by losing weight. You do not need a better reason to do it other than your desire to look good.

Eating is good for your health, and it keeps you healthy, but when you eat high-fat foods, and high carb foods, you could develop health problems, and you could get sick. What you want is to be healthy. When you are healthy, you are happy, and you can get new opportunities to be something you have always wanted to be.

Recipes

Almond Pancakes

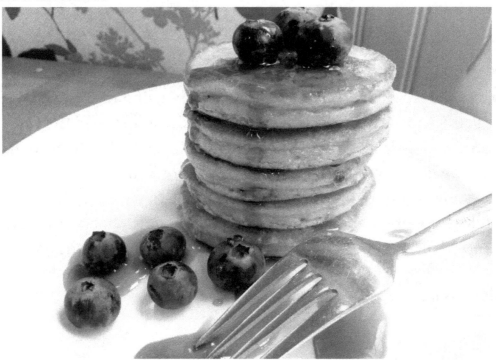

Preparation:4 min
cooking:6 min
servings:

Ingredients:

- ½ cup almond flower
- ½ cup cream cheese
- 4 eggs
- Cinnamon to taste
- Truvia to taste/vanilla extract
- Sides:
- 3 eggs

- Sea salt and pepper to taste

- 1 tablespoon grass-fed butter

- ¼ cup sugar free syrup

Directions:

1. Mix all ingredients in a blender until smooth

2. Spray nonstick cooking spray in a medium pan, fry remaining 3 eggs, season with salt and pepper, cook to desire doneness

3. Enjoy your pancakes (2 pancakes are enough for a meal) with butter, syrup and eggs on the side.

TIPS: if you like, add some crunchy bacon

Keto bread

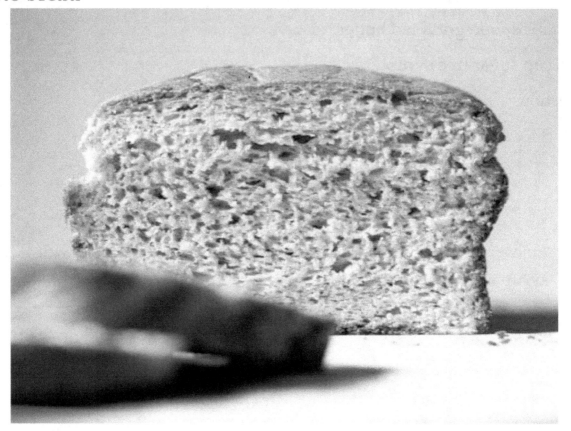

Preparation: 6 min
cooking:50 min
servings: 6

Ingredients:

- 5 tablespoons of psyllium husk powder

- 1 ¼ cups almond flour

- 2 teaspoon baking powder

- 1 teaspoon sea salt

- 1 cup water

- 2 teaspoon cider vinegar

- 3 egg whites

- 2 tablespoon sesame seed if desired

Directions:

1. Preheat oven to 350 F

2. In a bowl mix all the dry ingredients

3. Bring the water to boil

4. Add vinegar and egg whites to the dry ingredients and combine well, add boiling water and mix for 30 seconds until you have the consistency of play-doh

5. Shape 6 rolls and put on the oven tray, top with sesame seeds if desired

6. Bake on lower rack for about 50-60 minutes.Serve with butter or toppings of your choice

Jarlsberg Omelet

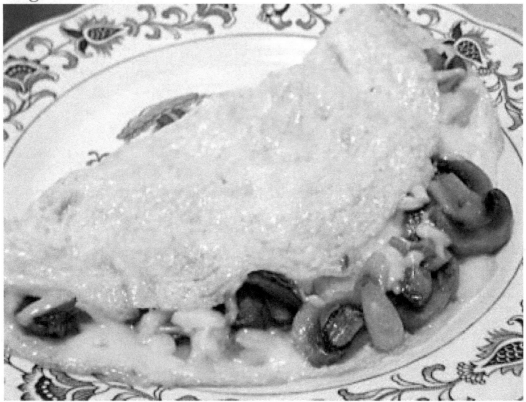

Preparation: 6 min

cooking:10 min

servings:1

Ingredients:

- 4 medium sliced mushrooms

- 2 oz. 1 green onion

- 1 tablesppon of butter sliced

- 2 eggs

- 1 oz Jarlsberg or Swiss cheese

- 2 slices of ham

Directions:

1. Cook the mushrooms the diced ham and the green onion in half of the butter in a big non-stick pan until the mushrooms are ready. Season with salt lightly, remove and set aside.

2. Melt over medium heat the remaining butter.

3. Add the beaten eggs

4. Now put the mushroom, ham and the grated cheese, on one side of the omelet.

5. Fold the plain side of the omelet over the filling once the eggs are almost ready.

6. Turn off the heat and leave until the cheese melts.

7. Enjoy it!

Crockpot Southwestern Pork Stew

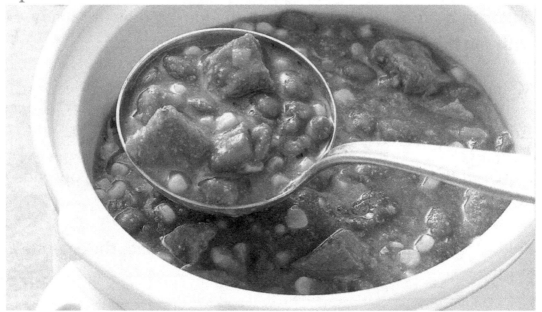

Preparation:10 min

cooking: 8 min

servings:4

Ingredients:

- 1 teaspoon of paprika

- 1 teaspoon of oregano

- 1/4 teaspoon of cinnamon

- 2 Bay leaf

- 6 oz. button mushrooms

- 1/2 Jalapeno

- 1 lb. sliced cooked pork shoulder

- 2 teaspoons Chili Powder

- 2 teaspoons cumin

- 1 teaspoon minced garlic

- 1/2 teaspoon Salt

- 1/2 teaspoon Pepper

- 1/2 Onion

- 1/2 Green Bell Pepper, chopped

- 1/2 Red Bell Pepper, chopped

- Juice from 1/2 Lime

- 2 cups bone broth

- 2 cups Chicken Broth

- 1/2 cup Strong Coffee

- 1/4 cup Tomato Paste

Directions:

1. Cut vegetables and stir fry on high heat in a pan. Once done, remove from heat.

2. Put sliced pork into the crockpot, add the mushrooms, bone broth, chicken broth, and coffee.

3. Add all the seasoning with the sauteed vegetables and stir well.

4. Cover the crockpot and cook for 4-10 hours at low temperature.

5. This recipe can be done with a cast iron boiler, the cooking time will be around 1 hour 20 minutes

Pan-Roasted Rib Eye Steak with Pan Jus

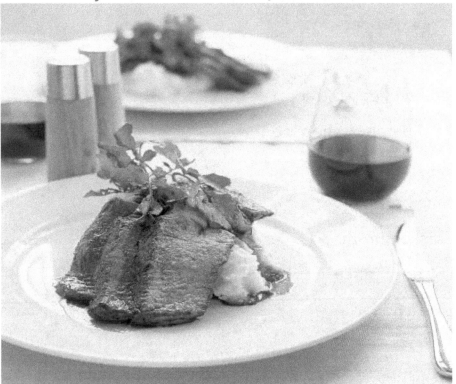

Preparation:45 min

cooking:20 min

servings: 3

Ingredients:

- 1 (1 pound) rib-eye steak

- 4 spoons of olive oil

- 1/2 cup Chicken Broth

- 3 spoons of room temperature butter

- sea salt and pepper to taste

Directions:

1. Before cooking, remove steak from the fridge for about 45 minutes, pat it dry, and salt it completely. Flip it through for about 20 minutes, remembering when flipping to pat it dry, and then again before cooking.

2. If you want to cook your steak medium or medium-well, preheat your oven to 200 ° F. Heat on the stovetop a cast-iron skillet or another pan over elevated heat.

3. Add the oil to the casserole.

4. Place the meat in the pan just before it starts smoking, then listen to the searing sound.

5. Leave it to cook for 3 to 5 minutes without shifting it.

6. Once the bottom has a pleasant brown color (you can check by lifting one edge of the steak to look at the bottom) flip over the steak and do the same on the other.

7. This will offer you a steak that is medium-rare. If you want to continue cooking, place medium-well in the oven at 200 ° F for 5 to 6 minutes and medium-well for 7 to 8 minutes.

8. Once done, put it on a cutting board for 5 minutes to rest.

9. Slice it and serve it.

10. Make the pan jus while the meat rests.

11. Transfer the pan to the stovetop, add the broth and water over medium heat, reduce the sauce by half, add the butter and stir from 2 to 4 minutes.

12. Pour the Jus over the meat and enjoy.

Conclusion

The ketogenic diet comprises a low-carbohydrate, high-protein and high-fat diet with a lengthy history of use in the management of intractable childhood seizures. Amid the existence of growing quantities of modern antiepileptic medications and surgical therapies, this nutritional therapy has enjoyed increasing success in recent years.

The authors study the past of the ketogenic diet, its conventional initiation protocol, potential modes of operation, proof of success, and side effects. In particular, several of the fields of an ongoing study in this area are illustrated, as are potential paths and unresolved issues.

An efficient and reasonably healthy cure for intractable epilepsy is the ketogenic diet. However, considering its lengthy past, everything regarding the diet, including its modes of operation, the optimum protocol, and the complete extent of its applicability, remains unclear. Diet study offers fresh insight into the causes underlying epilepsy and seizures itself, as well as potential possible approaches.

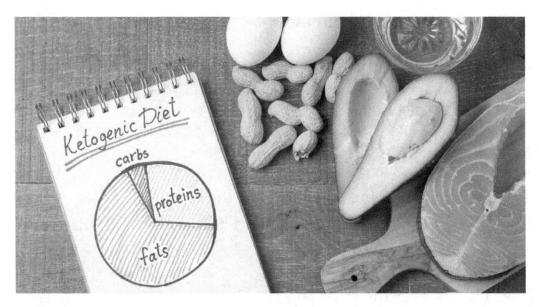

It would not be unreasonable to claim that when it comes to intermittent fasting, there is little to fear. While at first, you will feel starving, by triggering autophagy and losing more fat and ketones for food, your body will adapt.

A longer intermittent fast accompanied by shorter regular intermittent fasts is proposed by ketogenic diet researchers. In the days preceding and during the three-day fast, you will use a fasting regimen that involves fasting for up to three days, 3 to 4 times a year, with a shorter 10 to 18 hour fast.

If you are fasting for sixteen hours or three days to prevent symptoms of refeeding syndrome, checking your mineral levels is crucial.

To prevent unnecessary mineral depletion induced by ketogenic diets and fasting, supplementation of sodium from unprocessed potassium and salt, phosphate, and magnesium from mineral-rich foods or supplements could be essential.

 To put an end to it, it won't be wrong to say that the Ketogenic Diet is a miraculous diet as it focuses on healthy starvation and lets the body utilize the already stored fat and fastens the weight loss procedure as the intake of calories is less and the already stored fat is converted into energy by the body.

CPSIA information can be obtained
at www.ICGtesting.com
Printed in the USA
BVHW010944050821
613540BV00029B/373

9 781802 953800